NIGHT CLINIC

BY
DAVID GELBER

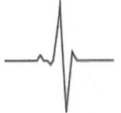

Ruffian Press
150 FM 1959
Houston, TX 77034
www.ruffianpress.com

ISBN-13: 978-0-9820763-9-2
ISBN-10: 0-9820763-9-8

First Edition – 2014

Typesetting/Book Layout Design:
Gianna Carini
www.brighteyes.org

Cover Design:
Courtney L. Gelber
http://www.courtneylgelber.com

Printed in the United States of America.

NIGHT CLINIC

BY
DAVID GELBER

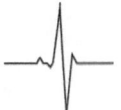

DEDICATION

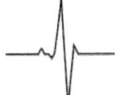

Night Clinic is dedicated to all my patients who have kept me up at night. They are all reminders of what it means to be a doctor.

INTRODUCTION

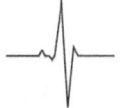

INSPIRATION POPS UP AT UNUSUAL TIMES AND IN THE strangest places. And so it came to be that "Night Clinic" was born in the wee hours of the morning while I was waiting to tackle a particularly nasty perforated colon. I was half dozing in the doctor's lounge at two in the morning, reclining on one of the couches, when my mind decided to wander away from the upcoming task of saving a life. My thoughts meandered their way towards speculation about all the doctors and nurses who regularly toiled throughout the night.

What type of patients go to the doctor at two in the morning?

Of course, there are the true emergencies, such as trauma or heart attacks, but there are also those individuals who live their lives between dusk and dawn, the denizens of the night.

Who are these people and what must a physician do to care for them? Prostitutes, addicts, insomniacs, criminals to name a few. But, what about the bizarre, the mystical, and the supernatural? Surely there are times when they need medical attention. Vampires and werewolves, dwarves, dragons, mythical beasts and magical beings pass through the doors of the Night Clinic to have their bodies, minds and souls mended and made whole after the day's toil. After all, even a superhero may need medical attention after battling the forces of evil in this world.

And so they come to the Night Clinic to be attended by intelligent, compassionate Dr. Barnes and intrepid, resourceful Nurse James. These two stalwart professionals care for their patients with a wink and smile, peppered with occasional outrage at the cruelty and injustice we all face in this world.

Each story stands alone, but they do build on each other until the final chapter. So come on in and check in with Miss James, let Dr. Barnes listen to your problems and your heart, and enjoy the wild and amazing ride on board the "Night Clinic" train.

Night Clinic

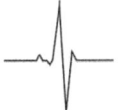

ANOTHER NIGHT IN THE FREE CLINIC; I'M NOT SURE IT'S worth one hundred an hour and it's a full moon. There'll probably be werewolves in every room.

"Dr. Barnes there's a patient in Room Two; infected leg, I think."

"Thank you, Miss James." *Nice legs,* I thought, staring at my assistant's shapely calves. *Keep your mind on work, Dr. Barnes.*

I opened the door and was immediately greeted by an overwhelming pungent force, a combination of month-old sweat, unwashed clothes, and rotting flesh. I called out into the hall: "Miss James, could you help me or send someone in here, please?"

"There's only me tonight, just a moment, Doctor," came the reply from down the hall.

I turned to the patient and tried to smile, while doing my best to keep my dinner down. "Mr. Smythe, I'm Dr. Barnes. What seems to be the problem?"

"It's these legs, Doc. Last month at the clinic they told me they was all healed, but now look at them." He smiled a broad smile revealing his three remaining teeth and bent over to roll up his pant legs. Crusted dirt fell to the floor. The pants would not roll up over his swollen limbs.

"You'll need to take them off," I suggested. *Where's that nurse or aid or somebody?*

I helped him unsnap the beltless pants and started to slide them down. He was wearing underwear, at least, although it was stained brown and tattered. As his trousers hit the floor they didn't crumple into a heap; instead, they almost stood up by themselves. His legs were just as I expected, swollen to three times normal size, colored a mixture of violet and brown with valleys of green black tissue, pus dripping from each wound. The ulcers on the left leg were cleaner, crawling with tiny maggots gorging themselves on the dead tissue, while leaving the healthy, vital tissue behind.

"Mr. Smythe, it appears your venous stasis ulcers have returned. How long have you had them?"

Mr. Smythe stroked his gray beard and a roach fell to the floor. "Well, I had those blood clots about ten years ago and ever since then my legs have been swolled up and these sores come and go."

I looked at his legs again. His thighs sported the healed scars of previous skin grafts. The ulcers had only minimal cellulitis and did not seem to extend to the fascia or muscle. At that moment the nurse came through the door.

"Miss James, I need to clean up these leg ulcers and we need some ethyl chloride for our little visitors here," I ordered while pointing to the maggot-infested wound on the left side.

Together we cleaned up Mr. Smythe's wounds, removing dead tissue, pus, and maggots. I debrided the right leg, while the maggots had done an excellent job on the left, leaving healthy pink tissue behind. We dressed the wounds with sterile gauze and offered to transport Mr. Smythe to the hospital for admission. He politely refused; we gave him a follow up at the wound care clinic, advised him to keep his legs elevated as much as possible, gave him enough gauze for a week of dressing changes, and the address to the nearest homeless shelter. He smiled as he left and I went on to my next patient.

Left breast pain; Evella, an unusual name, I thought as I marched through the door.

"Good evening, Miss Evella..." I started to say before I was interrupted.

"I am Evella, Goddess of the Night, young man," she exclaimed in a loud, melodious voice.

"I'm sure you are, Miss Evella," I replied in a flippant manner.

Sitting before me was a lady, mid-fifties, probably over three hundred fifty pounds, white hair on the right and jet black hair on the left, dressed in a skin tight black dress with a neck line that plunged to her navel, but covered by a sheer silk shawl. Despite this covering, her ample cleavage, along with tattoos depicting skeletons, angels, demons, and black snakes was clearly visible. The left breast didn't look right, even through the sheer covering. She smiled, revealing her tongue pierced by six gold rings and her top and bottom incisors fashioned into sharp fangs.

"OK, Miss Evella. It says you are having problems with your breast?"

"Please address me as Evella, Goddess of the Night, little man."

"Very well, Evella, Goddess of the Night, and I am **Dr. Barnes.** Now, how long has your breast been hurting you?"

"What does it matter to you, Doctor. It's obvious you don't really care. You look at me and think, 'Another crazy old woman; I'll try to be cordial.' Meanwhile your body language patronizes me more than your words and your eyes are already looking towards the door and your escape. You don't have to answer, Dr. Barnes, that look on your face has answered for you. Well, let's get on with it. My breast has been hurting for about six days. I tried Advil and warm soaks, but now it's red and swollen."

I looked into her eyes and then looked away, a bit embarrassed, not at the prospect of examining her breasts, more because she had figured me out so quickly and so completely, and called me out on it.

"Was it painful at first?" I asked.

"No, it was just red and swollen. The pain started to be really bad yesterday and I can hardly stand it. I tried some of these, but it only got worse."

She handed me a bottle of pills, Keflex, expired in 1998.

"How's your health besides this?"

"Oh, the usual, diabetes, high blood pressure, high cholesterol. Here's a list of my meds and allergies. Dr. Stanly Fried is my regular doctor."

I examined the list: Lipitor, Metformin, Metoprolol. Allergies to Codiene, Demerol, Dilaudid, Morphine.

"You're allergic to lots of pain meds. What happens when you take it?"

"Let's just say me and narcotic pain meds don't get along, Dr. Barnes. Aren't you going to check my breast?"

"Right away, Evella, Goddess of the Night. I'm just waiting for the nurse."

At that moment Miss James popped her head in. "Do you need any help, Dr. Barnes?" She smiled a broad smile and showed me a bit more leg than necessary.

"I need to examine the Goddesses' breasts. Could you get her ready? I'll be back in a minute."

I stepped out into the hallway, took a deep breath, waited about a minute and then stuck my head back into the room.

"She's ready, Dr. Barnes," Miss James informed me.

"Good, thank you," I answered. "Lay back and put your arm behind your head," I instructed the Goddess. I lifted the gown away to find a red edematous breast, skin dimpled, a hard mass in the axilla; clearly inflammatory breast cancer.

"How long has this breast been swollen, Evella, Goddess of the Night?"

"Maybe a few weeks. Is it something bad, Dr. Barnes?"

"It looks like what we call inflammatory breast cancer. Have you noticed this lump under your arm?"

"Not really," she replied. "Is it bad?"

"I can't say for sure without sampling the tissue, but it is almost certainly a type of cancer. You'll probably need chemotherapy."

I went on to explain the serious nature of her condition, that a biopsy would be necessary, and I gave her the name of an Oncologist at University Hospital, and I called him to let him know that she would be seeing him Monday morning. She thanked me for my time and disappeared into the night, clutching the paper with name of the Oncologist and the time of her appointment two days hence.

Are there two full moons tonight? Please make the next patient a sore throat. I picked up the chart outside the door to Exam Room Six: Edward Hyde, anal pain. Probably a thrombosed hemorrhoid. Finally something simple.

I knocked and then went into the room.

"Mr. Hyde, I'm Dr. Barnes. What seems to be the problem?" A middle-aged man stood in the corner, impeccably dressed with a brown derby on his head, black overcoat and pants, and fancy, black-polished shoes. He fidgeted a bit and had a distressed look on his face. *Must be a thrombosed hemorrhoid.*

"Pleased to meet you, Dr. Barnes," he answered with a slight British accent. "I have this sharp, throbbing pain in my bum, for five days now."

"Have you had pain like this before?" I asked, a routine question. "Any bleeding or swelling?"

"This is the first time, Doctor, no bleeding, but it feels as if my backside is the size of my hat. I suspect it's a thrombosed hemorrhoid. I have had some medical training as a doctor of sorts."

"Let's take a look, OK?"

He changed into a gown and I checked his backside which confirmed a single, thrombosed external hemorrhoid.

"You are correct, Mr. Hyde, or should I say 'Doctor,' a thrombosed hemorrhoid. I can remove that for you now if you wish."

"Thank you, Dr. Barnes."

I set up a procedure tray and slathered Mr. Hyde's swollen bottom with four percent lidocaine and took a ten-minute break while the lidocaine kicked in. Nurse James was in the break room smoking a cigarette.

"Those are bad for you, Nurse," I remarked.

"Oh, I know, but sometimes these nights get to me and I just have to have something to calm me down. I only smoke when I'm stressed out. Full moons always do it to me. I guess it's the werewolves."

"I haven't seen any werewolves, Miss James. We're in the middle of a city. Do you really believe there are werewolves out and about?"

"No doubt about it; there were four, no five, that came in last month. There was some big rumble between the vampires and werewolves and some of those boys were pretty beat up. Dr. Lyons spent five hours sewing them up."

"They didn't try to attack poor old Jack?"

"Well, they were a bit vicious at first, but five of Dilaudid and four of Haldol kept them quiet. We kept them locked up until the sun came up, they reverted back to their human forms and then they left quietly."

I put werewolves out of my mind as we left the break room to lop off Mr. Hyde's thrombosed hemorrhoid.

"OK, Mr Hyde, this might sting a bit," I warned as I cleaned the area around the hemorrhoid with some betadine. A purplish hemorrhoid the size of a jalapeño stared at me. I grabbed the syringe that was filled with lidocaine with epi then started to inject. I felt my patient tense up as I numbed the area, but beyond this normal response to my jabbing him with a needle, the area around the hemorrhoid changed. The skin became a bit darker and hair popped up on his buttocks. *Don't tell me he's turning into a werewolf.*

"Are you alright, Mr. Hyde?" I asked, but he only answered with a grunt.

"Miss James, is everything OK?" I asked again, a touch of worry in my voice.

"Vitals are normal, Doctor," she answered.

I grabbed the nasty hemorrhoid with a clamp and started to cut along its base. Halfway through there was a loud "BANG" and a crash.

"Mr. Hyde, what's gotten in to you?" Miss James yelled, her voice now filled with alarm.

Before I could finish snipping off the offending hemorrhoid, Mr. Hyde had jumped off the table and was flailing away with his walking stick, a heavy wooden staff with the head of a wolf sculpted into its top. I grabbed Miss James' hand and we raced out of the room. Shortly afterwards Mr. Hyde followed. Only he had changed. His face had grown long, unruly whiskers, his white teeth were now yellow and crooked, his hands had hair on the knuckles, and his manicured fingernails had become long and dirty. He was hunched over as he bolted out of the clinic and into the night.

"He should have less pain from that hemorrhoid, anyway," I concluded as I held up the clamp with the offending tissue held tight within its jaws. *Will this night ever end?* I went to the break room for a cup of coffee before seeing my next patient, a Mr. Pire, Chief Complaint: anxiety and suicidal ideation.

I glanced at Mr. V. M. Pire's chart before going into the room. The space for age was left blank, his vitals were: BP 60/30, heart rate 40, respiratory rate 12, temperature 92.

"Miss James, are these vitals correct," I asked, not believing the numbers.

"Took them three times, Dr. Barnes, but there's no need for alarm. You'll see what I mean when you see Mr. Pire," She answered in her most professional tone.

This night gets more bizarre every minute. I took a deep breath and let it out slowly, knocked on the door, and went in to see Mr. V. M. Pire. I saw a pale young man sitting on the chair in the corner, dressed in black pants, black shirt and wrapped in a black coat. Even with his coat he looked cold, shivering, his arms held tightly across his chest.

"Good evening, Mr. Pire. I'm Dr. Barnes. What brings you in here today?" I asked in my usual doctor's bedside tone.

"What's that supposed to mean? Do you think that I changed myself into a bat and flew in. Or maybe I just danced along the full moonbeam. I know what you're thinking: Another deluded, crazy who can't cope with reality," he spouted with venom in his voice.

"Actually, the way this night has been going, I was truly expecting a vampire. Who else could have vital signs like yours and not be in a coma? So tell me, what's the problem? If you don't want to say, you are free to leave. I have plenty of other sick people to attend to."

He calmed down, stood up, and started to pace around the room.

"I'm… I'm not sure where to start. You see, I… I've been having these fantasies and, well, with the full moon and everything, I just couldn't stand it. I even went to their meeting, thought about joining in their activities."

He paused for a moment. I could see he was upset and I tried to calm him down. I put my arm around him and lead him to the chair. He almost had tears in his eyes. "Go on," I said in a soft voice. "What are these fantasies?"

He looked at me with his dark, deep set eyes. "To be a wewuff," he whispered in a muffled voice.

"I'm sorry, I didn't understand what you said," I replied with true concern in my voice.

"To be a WEREWOLF," he answered loudly. "It's driving me crazy. I know it's ridiculous. I mean, I'm a vampire, the best of the best. Last month I downed six units of AB neg in under thirty seconds, all from the same vic… same donor."

"Sit down and tell me about it," I suggested, doing my best to imitate a Psychiatrist.

"I guess it started last full moon. I was out at night, like usual, and as I was flying around the neighborhood, thinking about dinner, I saw a whole pack of them, werewolves. They were circling around some helpless wino and then they attacked. After their kill they all howled at the moon, gave each other high fives, and then there were the girls. Dozens of them, all gathered around these vicious beasts, oohing and awing. Meanwhile, every night I'm out, shivering, looking for blood. Alone, hated by everyone, even other vampires who would just as soon cut your head off as share a drop of their precious stash."

"It must be a tough life," I observed.

"You don't know the half of it, Dr. Barnes. So, a couple of weeks ago, I'm laying in my coffin, trying to sleep. It must have been noon, and I start to thinking, *Wouldn't it be great to be a werewolf? Get to wear a fur coat, not be cold all the time, only worry about being a vicious monster once a month.* Then I say to myself, 'Get over it, you're a vampire, you're better than them.' But, I can't get over it; I can't get the thoughts out of my head. I tried to talk to one of the Elders. Well, you would have thought I was wanting to become a priest, the way he reacted. After that I got scared, I guess, and then I went to see them tonight. All the werewolves were gathered together, I even went inside, tried to meet them. As soon as they saw me they surrounded me. 'Look at sissy boy,' they taunted. 'Afraid of the big bad wolf?' I tried to talk to them, but they just laughed. I left, feeling more and more depressed. I just wanted to end it all. I even broke into the hospital and stole this."

He held up a case of thrombin.

"A couple of swigs of this, then all my blood congeals and it's the end. Well, I got scared and I wasn't sure what to do. I saw the Clinic sign and decided to stop in. So, here I am."

I stared at him for few moments, not sure what to say or do.

"Let me get you a blanket, you still look cold," I observed. "Stay here, I'll be back in a minute."

I stepped out into the hallway where Miss James was waiting.

"Dr. Barnes, you look a bit pale. Mr. Pire didn't attack you, did he?"

"No, Miss James, he only told me his troubles. I need to find the number to that Psychiatrist, the one that takes charity cases; Dr. Van Something…. Van Helsing. Here it is. Oh and I need a blanket and a couple of milligrams of Haldol, for the patient, not for me. Thanks."

I went back in armed with the blanket, a syringe filled with Haldol and Dr. Van Helsing's office number. I made a mental note to call Van Helsing later this morning and let him know about the referral.

"OK, Mr. Pire. I've got a shot for you that will help you calm down and here's the blanket I promised. Oh, and this is the number to a Psychiatrist I know. He'll take care of you for free. He does amazing work. After a few visits you'll forget that werewolves even exist. Now I need you to roll up your sleeve."

I gave him the shot and let him sit in the room for about thirty minutes, wrapped in the blanket. I definitely needed a few minutes alone after my visit with him and took refuge in the break room, drinking cocoa while Miss James took care of a baby with diarrhea and a teenage boy with a sprained ankle.

After finishing my cocoa I stuck my head into Mr. Pire's exam room and saw him sitting up, smiling, the blanket neatly folded on the exam table. He was holding his black jacket and, although still with a ghostlike pallor, he appeared to be in much better spirits.

"I feel much better, Doc. That shot really did the trick."

"I'll give you a prescription, Mr. Pire, and don't forget to call Dr. Van Helsing after nine this morning. I don't want to see you back here again."

"Thanks a lot, Dr. Barnes. It is a bit hard for me to call during the day, but I'll do what I can. Say, you don't happen to have any old pints of blood laying around, you know, a bag that might be expired that you're going to throw away anyway?"

"Sorry, we don't. Good night, Mr. Pire."

"No harm in asking. Good night, Dr. Barnes. See you around."

As he walked into the night, I heard a loud bang followed by howling.

"They're here, Dr. Barnes, worse than last month."

It was Miss James at the front door, which she had locked. Outside stood a half a dozen creatures, half upright, cloaked in brown and black fur, displaying long white fangs, deep red eyes and unpleasant dispositions. I looked at the clock, four a.m., still two and a half hours until it was light.

"Shouldn't we call the police?" She asked, fear in her voice.

"Take a close look, Miss James. They are the police."

The six monsters each had a shiny gold badge pinned to their fur and a few sported remnants of the blue police uniform. I thought for a moment and then turned to my frightened companion.

"Let them in, Nurse. We'll deal with them. Oh, do we still have that nitrous canister, you know, the one we use for little kids?"

Miss James smiled and replied in the affirmative.

"Could you please wheel it into Exam Room Eight; thank you."

We left the front door unattended, locked every Exam Room *but* number Eight with its door left ajar. I put some old food from the fridge, along with some bloody gauze bandages, in that room, opened the nitrous tank and let it flow. It wasn't long before the entire police force had broken in to our clinic and, following their noses, went straight into Room Eight. They attacked the food and the scent of blood made then even wilder. I quietly emerged from Room Seven and slammed the door to eight shut and locked it. After ten minutes the growling ceased. Miss James and I relaxed while we closed the clinic for the night and surveyed the damage. The front entrance was torn off its hinges, furniture upended and torn in the waiting room, and there were bloody stains on the floor and walls.

A short time later the sun came up and we let the town's police force out, and gave them paper gowns to wear home as they sheepishly emerged wearing nothing but their badges and slight grins. As they left I presented the Chief with a bill for the damage done, the cost of a tank of Nitrous Oxide, and use of the exam room for two and a half hours.

The day shift crew arrived thirty minutes later and Miss James I left together, went to PJ's Diner for breakfast, both of us vowing never to work Night Clinic during a full moon again. At least not until next month.

Another Night Clinic

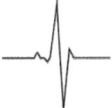

ANOTHER FULL MOON… ANOTHER NIGHT CLINIC. AT LEAST they fixed the front door and Miss James is with me again.

I walked through the main entrance and saw the new sign, "No Werewolves Allowed," handwritten in black and blue magic marker. *I see Miss James hasn't lost her sense of humor.*

"Good Evening, Miss James," I announced as I placed my backpack on the counter behind the nurse's station. "Are you ready for another action-packed full moon?"

"I'm ready, Dr. Barnes," she replied. "I've got my garlic, a crucifix, and a pack of silver bullets all right here in my pocket." She looked up from her desk and displayed a wide grin.

"That's just fine, Nurse, but, the garlic and crucifix are only for vampires and the silver bullets aren't much good unless they are used with a gun. No matter, I'm ready to get to work. Anything waiting?"

"Headache in Room Three."

Good, something simple.

I glanced at the chart. Twenty three years old, male, no significant past medical history. I knocked as I opened the door.

"Good Evening, Mr. Dallas. I'm Dr. Barnes. What is the problem that brought you here tonight?"

The patient was clean shaven with short brown hair and brown eyes; eyes which stared at me as I walked towards the exam table where my patient lay sprawled out. Those eyes looked up at me, filled with tears and fear.

"Oooh… uh… it's going to explode… Oo…" and his voice

trailed off and the eyes closed.

"Mr. Dallas, can you hear me?" No response. I grabbed his wrist and felt for a pulse... nothing. I punched the red emergency button on the wall as I felt for a femoral pulse, which was present but weak. Miss James burst through the door, crash cart in tow. I pulled the ambu bag from the wall and connected it to oxygen as Miss James hooked up monitors and handed me an endotracheal tube and laryngoscope.

Something simple?

"Tube is in," I exclaimed as I connected the ambu bag and began steady rhythmic squeezing.

"IV is in," Miss James countered.

I glanced at the monitor. Sinus Bradycardia with a rate of thirty. Miss James took over "bagging" Mr. Dallas while I made a quick surveillance. Left pupil reactive, right pupil dilated. No reaction to any stimuli, painful or otherwise. No sign of trauma anywhere. I picked up the red phone and called for an ambulance. Miss James continued ventilating our now relatively stable patient. His blood pressure was holding steady at 110/40, heart rate was now 50, and oxygen saturation was 100%. Two minutes later the ambulance arrived and Mr. Dallas was whisked away to County General Hospital for more definitive care.

"Another full moon?" Miss James commented rhetorically.

I just shrugged my shoulders. We went back to the break room to collect ourselves. I washed my hands and doused my face with cold water. Miss James took a drink of some Mylanta.

"Things like that always give me heartburn," she stated. "Give yourself a few minutes. All that's waiting is a simple... I promise... sore throat."

I sat at the table and fixed myself a cup of hot chocolate. Over the years I never could develop a taste for coffee. Tea was OK, but only after a fine meal, not at work. I perused the newspaper while I sipped on my cup and waited for my epinephrine level to fall.

Monarchs lost again, no surprise...government wants to raise taxes...

gang wars threaten to erupt…everything's depressing, nothing to give the average Joe hope. Oh well, time to get back to work.

I picked up the chart to Room One. Fourteen-year-old boy, Michael Drubitz, sore throat for two days, temp 101, everything else normal. I knocked on the door and walked in.

"Good Evening, Michael. I'm Dr. Barnes," I began with my usual introduction. I turned to the woman who was seated next to my patient. "Good evening, Mrs. Drubitz?" I asked, never assuming an adult with a child is the parent.

"I'm Sheila, Michael's mother."

"Pleased to meet you. What is the problem Michael is having?" I asked, turning to the young man.

"My throat hurts. I can barely swallow," the boy answered. I noticed he was flushed and he looked a bit listless.

"He started feeling sick three days ago at school. I kept him home yesterday and today. He had a fever of 104 this morning. He's had strep throat five times since January. He gets sicker each time."

"Let me have a look. Open your mouth wide, Michael."

I pushed on his tongue with the wooden tongue depressor and saw two huge tonsils, touching each other in the back of Michael's throat, yellowish exudates coated each one and the surrounding mucosa looked red and angry. A simple case of strep throat.

"It doesn't look too complicated, Mrs. Drubitz," A few days of antibiotics and he'll be up and around like nothing ever happened.

"Are you sure, Doctor? We never had anything like this until we came here," she observed. "At our old home, he never got sick."

"Changes always affect us. And the climate in this city seems to predispose to things like this," I responded, as I prepared the prescription for a Z-pack. He doesn't have any allergies, does he, Mrs. Drubitz?"

"Just to water," she answered.

"Excuse me, did you say 'water'?" I asked, more than a touch of disbelief in my voice.

"Yes, water," she answered in a matter-of-fact tone, as if it was a common condition.

"What happens if he is given water?" I asked with a bit of trepidation, wondering what I was getting myself into.

"Why, the same thing which happens to all of us," she replied.

"Which is…?"

"We get wet and then we melt," she replied.

"You melt?" *Why me?*

"Of course. It happens to all of us. I know you're thinking, 'She thinks she's some sort of wicked witch,' which I'm not, by the way. Let's just say that back home any contact with plain water has dire consequences. Look at this scar!" And she held up her hand to reveal a circular scar about two centimeters wide on her palm. "Drop of water fell there three years ago. Almost burnt a hole right through my hand. Luckily Michael here was able to get it off before it caused permanent damage."

"Just exactly where do you hail from, Mrs. Drubitz?"

She stared at her son for moment and then looked me in the eye.

"We're from, uh, Poland," she said.

"Uh huh," I murmured. "Well, Mrs. Drubitz, take the medication as prescribed. Does Michael have a family doctor or pediatrician?"

"Not really," she admitted.

"Here's the number to the Clinic at the University and also one for an Ear, Nose, and Throat specialist. He's had enough infections that he may benefit from consultation with an ENT to see if he needs his tonsils removed."

"Thank you so much, Dr. Barnes," she said effusively as she shook my hand. I noticed her hand was cold and felt a bit damp, like shaking the hand of a frog.

The two left, but as they were walking out I noticed that Michael had left what I thought was his cell phone on the exam table. I chased after them, but they were nowhere to be found.

Oh well, I guess they'll be back if they really want it.

I looked up and saw a bright shooting star at that very moment, racing away from the earth. It looked like it had just been launched from the park a few blocks away.

I wonder, nah, that can't be true.

I smelled my hand, the one that had shook Mrs. Drubitz' hand. It smelled of alcohol.

"Anyone else waiting, Miss James?"

"URI in two and diarrhea in four, and the Goddess of the Night dropped these off for you." She showed me a box of cookies thickly coated with powdered sugar.

"How is she doing anyway? She makes the best butter cookies."

"She looked good. Finished her first round of chemo. She said her breast is already better."

"That's great," I responded as I scarfed down four of the best cookies I'd ever had. I quickly dispatched the two waiting patients and sat down for a few moments to relax. My respite was short lived, however, as there were several loud shouts and I heard the door slam. We went out into the waiting room and found four teenagers lying prostrate in the waiting room. They were wearing gang colors and they were drenched in blood. Two were conscious and the other two were out, although both were still breathing.

"Just what we need," I blurted out, making no attempt to hide my exasperation. "Better call an ambulance."

"Right away, Doctor," Miss James replied.

At that moment there was a bright flash, followed by the loud boom of thunder, and then another and another. The lights flashed on and off, came back on for a moment and then went out.

"The phones are dead, Dr. Barnes," Miss James shouted, "and I can't get a signal on my cell."

I looked at my cell phone and saw the same thing: no signal. All of this transpired over a period of 30 seconds at the most. It was now pouring rain and we had only emergency lighting.

"We've got to do something fast for these two boys," I said, stating the obvious. I looked at the two conscious boys. One was holding his leg with a dirty towel which was drenched with blood, while the other had a handkerchief tie around his head and another around his left arm.

"You with the bandana," I screamed at the least injured of the four, "help me get your buddies into the exam rooms."

"I ain't doin nothing for those ugly 57's," he hissed with hatred in his voice. He jumped up and bounded out the door into the teeth of the torrential downpour.

One less bit of trouble, I thought, although I silently scolded myself for having such a thought. I turned my attention back to the other three problems at hand.

"Miss James, do you think we can get them into the exam room, at least."

I was down on the floor with one of them, feeling a very thready pulse, while my shapely companion was attending to the other, doing her best to check his blood pressure in the dim light.

"I think it's 70 over..."

At that moment there was a flash of blue light, short bang and a cloud of smoke, followed by the appearance of a man, dressed in tight black Spandex with a red "S" on the chest outlined by a hexagon of silver scalpels, wearing a tight black skullcap and a black surgical mask. He was solidly built with broad shoulders, bulging biceps and pecs, a six pack abdomen, and muscular thighs and legs. Miss James' jaw almost hit the floor when she saw him.

He was accompanied by a petite woman wearing a loose robe and a headband. She also sported a surgical mask, but hers was pulled down around her neck and she had a stethoscope around her neck and wide belt with many little compartments around her narrow waist.

"It's Captain Surgery," a booming disembodied voice announced.

"Da Da Da Daaaa..." an invisible band played.

"Stop with the music," Captain Surgery commanded and the music trailed away. "OK," he continued, "let's get these guys patched up."

"I suppose you're Lieutenant Flea?" I quipped.

"Cloud," she stated in a flat, deadpan voice.

"Dr. Cloud," the Captain added. "My trusted Anesthesiologist."

He then hoisted the two unconscious victims up above his head, one with each arm, while Miss James, Dr. Cloud, and I helped the third boy into one the exam rooms.

"Excuse me, uh… Captain, there isn't any power and there is no OR here; no lights, no nothing," I stated, trying to prevent starting up on something we couldn't finish properly. "Are you really a surgeon?"

He looked at me with his dark eyes which conveyed a sense of calm, intelligence and skill.

"Have faith, *Doctor*, Captain Surgery… (*Da da da daaaa*… he glared and the music stopped)… has been in much worse circumstances."

I saw him lay the first lad on the exam table. His eyes glowed as Dr. Cloud descended upon the boy's head. Captain Surgery started to glow with a purple light and when I looked back at the boy's head, he was intubated and being ventilated by Dr. Cloud. She had her finger on his temple and she began to speak loudly:

Heart Rate 140
BP 76/30
O2 sat 100%
Cardiac output 2 liters/minute
CO2 45

The Captains eyes continued to glow as he murmured, "Lacerated Liver, transected right Renal vein, transected peripheral nerve, perforated duodenum, approximately two liters of blood in the belly. OK, here we go."

I watched in awe as the black gloves he wore morphed from fingers to scalpel and clamps. A long incision was made. Sparks flew from the gloved fingers as each vessel was neatly cauterized and the incision carried deeper into the abdomen. Blood spewed forth and was expertly sucked up by a suction apparatus that had appeared from the belt around his waist. The blood was routed to the head of the table where it passed through a filter which was around Cloud's waist and then returned to the patient. I also saw antibiotics infuse along with fluids and various anesthetic agents. All the time Cloud never took her finger off his temple and continued to rhythmically announce physiologic parameters.

Captain Surgery worked in near silence, only a rare murmur escaped from his lips. His eyes glowed and emitted light which illuminated the field in the darkened room. As he ran his fingers over the abdominal structures he mumbled each by name.

"Liver segment four lacerated with bleeding branch of hepatic artery and portal vein."

Flashes of light and wisps of smoke emanated from the surgical field as his fingers danced over the injured organs at lightning speed.

"Vessels sealed, hemostasis achieved," he announced. "Renal vein repaired and the kidney remains well perfused and functional. Duodenum repaired and buttressed. Final scan, all injuries addressed."

A torrent of clear fluid flooded out of his left hand as the abdomen was irrigated.

"Time to close," he announced.

I watched as he ran his hand up and down the wound which left the fascia closed. He infused a blue fluid into the wound and then ran his hand along the wound again, closing the skin. Finally, a clear fluid was applied and then dried, sealing the wound closed. The entire surgery had lasted only about 12 minutes.

"He'll be good as new in a few hours," the Captain announced. "On to the next victim, I mean, patient."

He went to the next table, once again eyes glowing as he scanned the patient. Cloud had the patient asleep in seconds and began her litany of vital signs and physiologic parameters.

"Look bad, Captain?" I heard her ask. "BP is forty."

"Two gunshots; colon, superior mesenteric artery, just missed the spinal cord, second bullet went through the small bowel and right kidney. But, Captain Surgery… (*Da, da,* another glare from the Captain's eyes and the music stopped abruptly)… is on the case."

Once again the violet light engulfed his body and he went to work, his eyes shining, his fingers dancing, blood splattering here and there and then… silence, a few flashes of light, and he started to close.

"BP's ninety, Captain, heart rate's down to ninety five and oxygen delivery is normal. Great save."

"Thank you, thank you," the Captain said with a bit of humility. "now on to the final lad."

This time Cloud ran her hand across the patient's abdomen which numbed him from the waist down. Captain Surgery reached his hand towards the gunshot wound, made a clean incision which exposed the injured artery. The index finger from his left hand deftly encircled the artery above the injury while his left fifth finger controlled the distal artery. His right index finger ran up and around the injured segment and, when he was finished, left the artery perfectly repaired with an excellent, bounding pulse. He ran his right hand up and down the open wound and then pulled it out. The swelling disappeared and the wound sealed itself up.

"All three of these fine young men should be up and around in a few hours, Doctor. Have them follow-up at the University Clinic next week. They've received antibiotics and have been infused with extended pain relief. Well, Cloud, our work here is done. Wherever there is injury and disease, Captain Surgery… (*Da, da, da, daaaaa*)… will be there."

"Always the dramatics," Cloud whispered to Miss James.

"Did you say something, Dr. Cloud?" the Captain asked.

"I said you're a virtuoso," she replied. "It's a living," she remarked as she packed up all her equipment.

At that moment the lights came on, the three gang members were all up and walking around and I saw a white light emanate from the Captain, which left his black, spandex outfit spotless. Every speck of blood and fluid washed away.

"Uh, Captain," I asked, "shouldn't you have a cape?"

"No capes, no capes; nothing but a nuisance, getting caught in doors, dragging on the floor, and picking up all sorts of loose debris and germs. And, do you know how expensive they are to clean?"

He paused for a moment.

"Now remember, if you suffer from serious injury, broken bones, ruptured colons, ulcers, gallstones, hemorrhoids, cataracts, ear wax build-up, or, well you get the idea. Just whisper my name, Captain Surgery *(Da, da, da, daa)* and I'll be there."

There was a flash of light, a puff of smoke, and they were gone.

"Do you believe that, Miss James? Vampires, werewolves, and now this. I don't think they pay us enough. That Captain Surgery… *(Da, da,da, daaa)*… is quite remarkable. "

Miss James let out a big sigh. "I hope he comes back." And, she sighed again.

"Muscles, brains, and superpowers are not everything, nurse," I commented. *Then again, maybe they are.*

"Look at the time; this shift is almost over. Anyone else waiting?"

"No, Dr. Barnes."

"Good, I could use some breakfast."

And we left together as the day shift arrived.

MORE NIGHT CLINIC

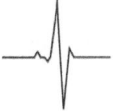

"I DON'T KNOW WHY I'VE COME BACK," I STATED TO NO one in particular. "Werewolves, vampires, aliens, super hero surgeons; why can't we have a nice quiet night clinic for once. You know, a sore throat, sprained ankle, maybe a little diarrhea."

Miss James stared at me and then gave me that smile, the one that says, "You're sort of cute, but I think trouble follows you." I smiled back, sheepishly.

"At least there isn't a full moon tonight; just the opposite, new moon and foggy," she announced. "I think it will be slow, for once. Nobody's come in yet."

"That's fine, Miss James. I've got Grand Rounds this weekend anyway. Maybe I'll have the chance to bone up on parasitic diseases of North America. Can you believe it? We see heart disease, cancer, trauma by the boatload, and Dr. Weiss wants me to talk about worms and fleas."

"Cheer up, Dr. Barnes, you won't be a resident forever."

I gave her a frosty look which only made me look silly and then announced I'd be in the call room if she needed me. I was deep into the life cycle of the deer tick when the phone rang.

"Per your request, there is diarrhea in Exam Room Two."

"Thank you, Nurse. I'll be there in a few minutes."

I'm bored with studying anyway.

I picked up the chart on the door. Six-year-old boy, diarrhea for three days, no fever, heart rate 100, BP normal.

At least it doesn't look like cholera.

"Good evening, Mrs... Cichello," I announced, glancing down

at the chart. "Did I pronounce that right?"

"Quite so Dr…"

"Oh, it's Barnes… Dr. Barnes. Now what seems to be the problem?" I asked with my very serious professional tone.

"Andrew has been sick since Monday," she announced. "He started with fever and then he vomited four… no five times, and now he is having diarrhea."

I looked at the boy. His cheeks were a bit flushed, but he looked alert and certainly was not in any severe distress. Then I looked at Mrs. Cichello. She had on full length leather coat with some sort of fur making up the collar. She had a large diamond ring on her left hand and an even larger emerald ring on her right. She was carrying a Chanel bag and her wristwatch was studded with diamonds. Still, she seemed a bit unsettled to me. She glanced at the door to the Exam Room several times and then looked down at her watch.

Probably has a date or something. I wonder where the servants are hiding?

As if she were reading my mind, Mrs. Cichello announced, "Such a bother and on Marie's night off."

"Excuse me?" I asked.

"Marie, little Andrew's nanny, is off on Thursdays. It's such a bother."

"I'm sure it is," I replied and then I turned to Andrew. "Can you climb up on my table here, Andrew?"

In a flash the boy was sitting on the exam table. I went through the usual questions and obtained a perfect history for Rotavirus. The boy's abdomen was benign and his temperature and all other vital signs were normal.

"I think Andrew just has a bit of a virus, Mrs. Cichello," I explained. Just make sure he drinks plenty of fluid and he should be back to his old self in a few days."

"So you think he's well enough to come home? How can you be sure he doesn't have appendicitis? Oh, I knew I should have taken him to a real hospital."

"I can assure you, Mrs. Cichello, he'll be fine."

"This can't be. I know it's something serious. I'll bet he's got food poisoning, probably *Salmonella*. Dr. Barnes, if you send him home I know something terrible will happen. Why there's no question but he should be in the hospital. Oh, why do such things have to happen when Marie is off?"

I was starting to wonder more about Mrs. Cichello. A mother would normally be relieved when told that her son did not have a serious illness, but this mother was anxious for her son to be sick enough to be hospitalized. I put two and two together and asked, "Why don't you want your son at home, Mrs. Cichello?"

At first she gave me a look of feigned indignation and she started to raise her voice, but I held up my right index finger, sort of a signal for her to stop. She glanced at the Exam Room door again and then opened her purse and fumbled for her wallet.

"I don't want any of your money, just tell me the truth."

"Well, it's just that my club is meeting at my home tonight and I don't have my usual help and Andrew being sick. I thought that maybe he should be in the hospital."

I looked at Andrew and then at his mother. I felt no pity for his heartless mother, but I did feel for the boy.

"Let me take another look at him," I said softly. I gazed into his eyes and felt his tummy again, moved his head back and forth.

"Well, I think it might be best to watch him for a few hours. I think we should keep him here, until, say, midnight; just to be on the safe side."

"Thank you, Dr. Barnes. I'll pick him up by 12:30."

"Goodnight, Mrs. Cichello," I said. "Make sure we have your number in case Andrew takes a turn for the worse."

She gave me an indignant look and then left, closing the door with a bit more force than necessary.

"Looks like it's you and me and Miss James, Andrew. You can wait in the break room. Miss James will find you some games or something to keep you from being bored."

"I think I'd like to lie down for a while," he answered.

"OK, OK, you can have my call room."

I fixed him up in my room and then returned to work.

The next few hours brought a steady stream of vomiting drunks, sniffles, and minor injuries. Nothing very exciting and nothing very taxing. Miss James and I checked on Andrew every twenty or thirty minutes; he seemed to be content just sitting in my room, playing games on the computer or drawing pictures with the magic markers and paper Miss James had scrounged up.

It was now after midnight and I was expecting Mrs. Cichello to walk through the doors at any moment. We had finished with the last patient and there was a brief lull. Instead of Mrs. Cichello, it was a street lad named Daniel who walked through the door.

He was in Exam Room Two and the chart said, "Chief Complaint: Bald Patches." The rest of the chart was blank; the spaces for date of birth, address, phone number, and everything else were all empty. I wasn't sure what to expect as I knocked on the door. Seated on the floor was a boy, perhaps eight years old and holding a dog of no particular breed. The boy was dressed in a filthy gray coat, his blondish hair had a mind of its own as it stuck out in every direction, he wore dirty, torn jeans and tennis shoes which were also dirty and worn with frayed laces which didn't match. His eyes, however, were another story, big and blue, full of curiosity and sensitivity. The dog growled at me as I walked in and I immediately noticed several bald patches on the mutt, with some sores which were a mixture of dried blood and dead skin.

"If your companion wants to be seen, I suggest he stop growling at his doctor," I remarked. "I'm Dr. Barnes, young man. You are Daniel?"

He stood up and held out his hand before speaking, softly, "I'm Daniel and this is Becky. She's sick."

"You know this isn't a veterinarian clinic, Daniel, and I'm not a veterinarian."

He looked down at the floor and then replied, "I know, but

some of the others said you were a good guy. I waited three days until I saw you were working. Please, Dr. Barnes, can't you just look at her?"

Daniel gave me a big smile and then picked Becky up and held her to his chest.

"OK, OK, let's take a look. I'm not guaranteeing I'll do anything, but... what's this?" I asked as I gazed at the bald patch on the mongrel's neck. I pinched a spot at the edge of the bald patch and looked between my fingers. "*Ctenocephalides canis* I believe, otherwise known as a flea. As a matter of fact, she's got lots of fleas."

I ran my fingers along Becky's back and three little black bugs jumped off. I quickly gathered them up in a Kleenex and flushed them away.

"I would say that Becky here needs a flea bath as the first step in her treatment. Unfortunately, flea shampoo is something we don't usually keep here in the clinic."

"I could go out and steal some," Daniel volunteered.

I gave him a false stern look, before remarking, "I think we can buy some, but not at this hour. Maybe there's some sort of home remedy for fleas."

We looked at the computer together and found a few different home remedies. One was plain old Ivory soap.

"Well, Daniel, let's give her a bath. Wait, I'll get some help."

I found Andrew sleeping in my break room, his head cradled on my textbooks. *Probably the best use for those books*, I thought as I gently roused him.

"What... wha, is my mom here?" he asked as he sat up rubbing his eyes.

"Not yet, but I need your help; I need you to help give Becky a bath."

"I can't give a bath to some old girl," he protested.

"Come on, you'll see," and I motioned for him to follow me.

Well, his eyes lit up when he saw the dog and he and Daniel got down on their knees and scrubbed Becky from nose to tail. I saw some fleas fall off and wash away down the drain. Becky, to her credit, stood like a statue as the two boys scrubbed and combed and scrubbed some more.

While the two boys were occupied I had to attend to a few sick patients, a sore throat in a four-year-old girl and a laceration to the arm in a man who decided to hang some pictures at 2:00 a.m. Miss James brought some towels for Becky was the boys finished washing her down. Of course, she had to shake herself dry first, giving Daniel and Andrew a good washing, as if they needed any more. Miss James helped dry all three of them.

After the bath I gave Becky a closer inspection. I was no veterinarian, but I had always had a dog up until I started medical school. Her teeth were white and intact, I estimated she was pretty young, no more than two years old, probably younger. Although she was thin with all the bald spots, she otherwise looked to be in pretty good health.

The bald spots were red in some spots and there was some drainage which was yellowish. I decided to treat them as burns. I pulled out a large jar of Silvadene cream and told the boys to put it on the Becky's bald spots, like they were icing a cake. As they were finishing, Mrs. Cichello finally made her return. It was 2:30 in the morning.

"You're a little late, Mrs. Cichello."

"I guess I lost track of the time. Is it really after two? You know how girls can be when they get together."

She seemed to be nervous, looking over her shoulder at the parking lot, as her facial expression alternated between a forced smile and worry.

"Please, I just need to pick up Andrew and then you'll never see us again." She glanced over her shoulder again.

"OK, just follow me. He's feeling much better, by the way. I thought you'd want to know."

"Oh… really? That's great. You must be a really fine doctor. I thought for sure he'd end up in the hospital."

I brought her into Exam Room Three just as the two boys were finishing dressing Becky's wounds. Both boys had as much Silvadene on themselves as they'd managed to get on the dog.

"We need to go now, Andrew," Mrs. Cichello commanded, her voice carried an abrupt edge and more than a touch of worry.

"Just let me get cleaned up and then we can go," Andrew replied. He went to the sink and started to wipe away the white cream.

"Now, young man," she said even more forcefully.

Becky started to growl and then the door to the exam room flew open.

"I'm tired of waiting, bitch," a heavy set man screamed as he grabbed her by the arm. He grabbed her and Andrew and started out the door when there was a loud, deep bark, a growl, and then flurry of Silvadene and canine as Becky jumped on the neck of the man. Mrs. Cichello managed to break herself and Andrew free as that little dog showed just how ferocious a street mongrel could be.

Daniel, demonstrating some of his survival skills, started pulling the man's hair. The man tried to reach around and pull his attackers off, but both Becky and Daniel were tenacious. In the midst of all this excitement Miss James stepped out, returning a minute later with a syringe filled with something which she jabbed into the man's leg as he struggled to pull Becky and Daniel off.

After a few minutes he quieted and Daniel gave a short whistle. Becky left the man alone and returned to her master's side.

"A little Thorazine and Morphine works quite well," Miss James announced.

I called the police while Mrs. Cichello stood in the corner cradling Andrew. Daniel sat on the floor with Becky, dutifully reapplying the Silvadene cream which was now smeared all over him, the room, and the would-be attacker.

"What is it all about, Mrs…" I started to ask.

"Please, call me Lucia," she said before I could ask for more details. "That is Cosmo, hired help. It's pretty complicated. Let's just say it has a something to do with drugs and smuggling and kidnapping and I'm, no we, were in big trouble. That's why I left Andrew here and that's why I'm so late picking him up. I kept trying to figure out some way to stop what was happening."

The police arrived at that moment and Cosmo, still out like a light, was handcuffed, loaded on a stretcher, and carted away. I started to say something to the officer, but Lucia shook her head and then she spoke.

"Officer, I had left my son here to be observed because he was ill and Dr. Barnes thought he might need to be in the hospital. My boy, however, is much better and so I came to pick him up. That hooligan followed me in here and broke into the exam room demanding drugs. He would have gotten away, too, except for this little boy and his dog. They saved the day."

The police took down everyone's name and contact information and then went on their way. After all the excitement, I took a seat in the waiting room with Miss James and Mrs. Cichello.

"OK, Lucia, what's this all about. Certainly not that fairy tale you told the police. The way things seem to happen around this clinic, you're probably some sort of international spy caught up in espionage with the fate of the world hanging in the balance. Or, you're really a vampire and you've been out hunting up victims to feed your son."

Mrs. Cichello looked at me and then at Miss James. She straightened her designer jacket and started to speak:

"Dr. Barnes, I am certainly no spy nor am I a vampire or any other sort of monster. I was involved with some bad, dangerous people from Mexico, but that is all over now. With the local police involved and Cosmo in custody, I don't think I'll have any more problems."

"Are you sure? Some of these crooks can be pretty vengeful, at least that's what I've heard."

"Trust me, I'm sure. Just bring me Andrew and we'll be on our way."

Miss James went to get the boy while his mother sat silently.

Finally, she spoke.

"I love him more than anything, you know, Andrew, that is. That's why I left him here this evening, to keep him safe. I'm sure you thought I was or am a terrible mother, but I really was trying to keep him out of harm's way. Please don't ask me anything else; just believe that everything is fixed and neither Andrew nor myself are in any danger."

"If you say so. I'm just a hired gun here at the clinic. I certainly do not want to be involved in any Mexican drug wars, smuggling, or kidnapping."

At that moment Miss James returned with Andrew, Daniel, and Becky.

"Time to go, Andrew," Lucia announced.

Andrew hesitated for a moment. "What about Daniel and Becky? Where are they going to go?"

Lucia looked at the two orphans. "I'm sure Daniel's mother is worried…"

"Daniel doesn't have a mother, nor a father or any family, Lucia," I informed. "He lives moment to moment on the streets, like too many others. Why do you think this clinic is here? There are a lot more like Daniel out on the streets."

"Can't Daniel stay with us, please?" Andrew asked, his eyes pleading. "I helped him with Becky and we got to be good friends."

Lucia stared at the thin boy and then at Becky, letting out a smirk at the sight of the dog and her patches of white Silvadene cream.

Andrew added, "Mom, you know how you always give me things, toys and stuff to play with? And, you know I take them and play with it for a few minutes? But a lot of the time I bring those toys to school with me and give them to other kids. And you what? I feel much better giving the toys away than getting them. I think I'd like to give my room to Daniel and Becky. Can't I do that, Mom, please?"

Lucia smiled, first at her son, then at me, and finally at Daniel.

"What do you say, young man? Would you like to come stay with us? And Andrew doesn't even have to give up his room, we've got an extra bedroom for you and Becky."

Daniel smiled from ear to ear, a clear answer to everyone present. The four of them walked out together. The sun was releasing its first rays of the day as they piled into a black Mercedes and drove away.

"I'm not sure we should let you moonlight here anymore, Dr. Barnes," Miss James remarked. "You bring too much excitement."

"I thought it was you, Miss James. Come on. It's quitting time. I'll buy you breakfast."

Months later I did learn more about Lucia and Andrew. Although there were some sketchy reports in the papers, it was only after I ran into them walking in the park that I learned the truth.

Lucia was married to the CEO of a big Mexican drug manufacturer, but was separated from her husband and trying to get a divorce, something about his being abusive and a number of mistresses. That fateful night, she had gone, supposedly, to meet her husband and settle things once and for all. Unfortunately, her husband had sent Cosmo who followed her to the clinic and was trying to force both of them back to Mexico. As it was, her husband had been arrested and now she was safe with Andrew, Daniel, and Becky, whose fur had grown back beautifully.

Footprints Across Night Clinic

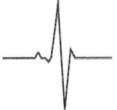

"ANOTHER SATURDAY NIGHT, ANOTHER STINT IN THE night clinic," I muttered as I snuck in the back door. *I wonder what adventures await Miss James and me tonight?*

"Good evening, Doctor," an unfamiliar voice greeted me.

"Hello, uh… where's Miss James?" I asked the heavy set woman dressed in white. I think she sensed my disappointment.

"I'm sorry, Dr. Barnes," she replied, her voice sporting an edge that said I know I'm not young and blonde and shapely, but I do know my job. "Miss James asked me to cover for her. She had to go out of town suddenly; something about her twin sister and a rash and fever. Anyway, she's not here. You'll just have to get by with frumpy old Maggie."

"Pleased to meet you frumpy old Maggie; I'm chastised young Dr. Barnes. Anything waiting for me?"

"There's one patient left over from the day shift, older man with pus draining from his penis. I guess Dr. Wacker didn't have time to get to him."

I picked up the chart. Fifty-five… no address… arrived at… "Three o'clock? Maggie, what's the deal? He's been here for five hours."

"I guess they were busy."

I shook my head and wondered how busy they really had been, then shrugged my shoulders and turned to face the problem at hand.

"Well, I guess I'm off into the world of pus-sy penises. If I'm not out in five minutes, page me."

I knocked on the door and then entered. Seated on the chair was a very large naked man with a paper sheet over his groin. A large pannus hung down almost to his knees.

"Good evening, Mr. Jonas. I'm Dr. Barnes. What seems to be the problem?"

"Well, it's about time. The problem? Can't you see it? I think it's about to fall off."

"What's about to fall off?" I asked, trying to sound concerned.

"Why, my gentils. Burning and dripping for days. I knew I never should have gone."

"Gone where?"

"Upstairs at the Palace. I knew I'd catch some disease."

"When did you go to the Palace?"

"Let's see, it was Tuesday, no Wednesday."

"So, you went to the Palace three days ago?"

"Three days ago? No, no, no, doc. It was, let me think, Wednesday, June 3rd, 2010. I just knew that whore would give me the clap."

"Mr. Jonas. If it's been three years since you went to the Palace, I don't think your problems have anything to do with catching the clap from any lady that you might have encountered."

"It has to be that. I haven't been to any hookers since."

"Just tell me when everything started."

"Well, it was on a dare. Some of my quote... *friends*... unquote said I didn't have the balls to go, pardon my pun. Well I proved them wrong. I went and now look at me."

I did look at him and then asked, "you mean that you have all these symptoms you are suffering?"

"No, no, look at how big I've become. Back in twenty ten I only weighed a hundred and eighty. Now I must be four hundred..."

"At least," I observed. *This could go on for hours.* "Tell you what, let me take a look at your problem and I'll see what I can do. Can you lie down on the table so I can examine you?"

"OK, Doc." He pushed down on the table a couple of times, checking to see if it was sturdy enough and then slowly climbed up and lay down. His large belly hung down over the area in question.

"Uh, do you think you can hold your belly up?" I asked gingerly, trying to be at least a little tactful.

"Oh, sure."

Beneath the massive pannus, which was edematous and red, I saw a small, retracted penis and scrotum. After much digging, I managed to get a proper hold of it and examined it. There was purulent drainage emanating from a remnant of foreskin and the suprapubic area was ulcerated secondary to irritation from his huge apron of a belly.

"I don't think your encounter at the Palace is responsible for your current problem, unless you want to count your guilt at having frequented that establishment. No, the problem you are having is that your belly is too big and it looks like you're having trouble keeping yourself clean. Do you have any help at home?"

"Just my mother, but she will let me have it if she finds out I've been to see one of those whores at the Palace."

"Well, you really don't need to tell her. However, can she help clean you up? I think if you get in the shower and clean yourself well, and then apply one of the medicated patches I'm going to prescribe, you'll be better in no time."

"We can give it a try. Mother will do whatever is necessary. It's what mother's are for."

I nodded my head and called for Maggie. The two of us cleaned him up and dressed the open wounds, which were actually pretty clean, with Duoderm dressings. I gave him a prescription for some antibiotics to treat what appeared to be cellulitis of his huge pannus and a follow up appointment at the family practice clinic at the University hospital, attention to Dr. Wacker.

Revenge can be so sweet.

"What's next Maggie?" I inquired as I rubbed my hands with the waterless cleaner which hung on the wall at strategic points throughout the clinic.

"Back pain for three years in Room Three, lacerated arm in 4, and a burn to the hand in Five."

"Is it bad, the burn to the hand, I mean? Because, if it is, then we might as well just call the Burn Unit now."

"Second degree at worst. You should be able to handle it."

I nodded my head and then went back to the supply closet to get a new box of gloves. As I walked I noticed some peculiar footprints on the floor.

"Maggie, did you notice these footprints? It looks like some wild animal has been walking around."

The footprints were very unusual. They were a cast of dirt and grease, three toes with long claws which looked like the perpetrator walked for a short ways, then jumped to the end of the hall where there was a water fountain, and then jumped back, where there were some more footprints leading nowhere in particular.

"Very strange, Dr. Barnes, very, very strange."

"I guess there's no time to worry about it now," I remarked, believing that one of the patients or personnel from the previous shift had brought their dog to work. It wasn't long before I found out how wrong I was.

I checked on the burned hand first.

"Hey, Doc," a familiar voice called out.

"Vince? What are you doing here at this hour?" It was Vince Smialdi, one of the maintenance workers for the clinic.

"Well, you know, Doc, I was in the back checking out the store room. I thought I smelled some smoke back there. Anyway, I was in the store room and I found this. What do you make of it?"

He held up what appeared to be half of a large golden eggshell, broken and burned at the edges. The shell was at least twelve inches wide.

"Looks like one of the proverbial golden eggs, but I'd hate to get cornered by the goose that laid it," I observed.

"That's what I thought. Looks like a giant egg shell, but it's only gold color. Look…"

He grabbed some of the broken edge and broke a piece off. It was brittle, just like any eggshell.

"A mystery, that's for sure," I replied.

Could this have anything to do with those footprints?

"Uh, Doc."

I looked up from my thoughts and saw Vince with a perplexed look on his face.

"Oh, sorry, Vince. I was just thinking. Maggie and I saw some unusual footprints in the back. It wouldn't surprise me if the two were somehow related. But first, let me look at your hand."

He held up his right hand. The palm was red with large blisters.

"I got this when I picked up that eggshell. It was like picking up the business end of a branding iron. I rinsed my hand in some cold water, but after I got home those blisters popped up, so I came back here to the clinic."

"A good thing, too, although this isn't terrible. Second degree at most. Let me dress it for you and then you can be on your way. No, on second thought, why don't you stay for a bit, if you don't mind. Maybe, you and I, we can investigate some of these strange things: this eggshell and those footprints. You don't mind, do you? Let me finish up with the patients who are waiting and then we can check things out."

"No problem, Doc. I don't have anyone at home anyway."

Vince had been alone for years. His wife had passed away and both his kids had moved and lived on the west coast.

I left him in the break room and went back to my patients. I gave the back pain a shot, stitched the laceration, but then had to deal with a cocaine overdose, a baby with a fever, a broken arm, two hookers who got into a fight over a "customer" and a drunk woman who had pneumonia after passing out, vomiting, and aspirating. I had to wait for an ambulance to ship her to the County.

It was 3:30 a.m. when I was finally free. I found Vince sleeping on the sofa.

"How's the hand?" I inquired, making small talk as we ventured to the back of the clinic. I left Maggie up front to man the fort should any patients arrive. On most nights business slowed considerably after about 2:30 a.m. The bars were closed, everyone who was going to hook up had done so. Sick kids and their worried parents had fallen into fitful slumber. It was the time I usually managed to grab a couple of hours sleep. Tonight, however, I was a sleuth, investigating a deep, dark mystery.

Sometimes my imagination gets the best of me.

Maggie had cleaned up the tracks by the supply room, but I saw fresh ones near the storage closet. There was a faint scent, like burned plastic.

"Do you think it's safe," I asked, grabbing Vince by the arm. "What do you think is in there?"

My thoughts drifted back to werewolves, vampires, aliens, and so many other bizarre things I'd encountered here at the clinic.

"Don't worry, Doc," he replied, trying to reassure me. "Two to one it's an ostrich or something like that."

Just to be on the safe side I picked up a broom that was in the hallway.

"That's great. If there's some sort of monster you can sweep it under the table. You're not much for adventure, Doc."

"If I want excitement, I'll go to an amusement park. I'm just an old country doctor, to quote Dr. McCoy."

Vince picked up a flashlight as he slowly pushed the door to the storage room open. It gave a loud squeak. I thought I heard some fluttering noises. Vince shined his light to the back of the room, starting at the floor and up to the ceiling.

"There, see them? More footprints. They lead to that back corner."

He slowly made his way towards the footprints, while I followed closely behind, clutching the handle of the broom, its bristles out in front of me, ready to swipe at whatever vicious brute was waiting out there, surely ready to pounce on us.

We made it to the back of the room. There were greasy footprints all over, but nothing else. Vince shined his light in every corner, but saw nothing. It was at that moment I glanced up and saw the faint silhouette of something hovering in the corner, wings beating against the air. There was a faint glow from two deep red eyes and then flames shot out towards the two of us. I grabbed Vince and pulled him down to the floor as a white hot stream of fire shot across the room, leaving smoke and a blackened wall where the flames had hit.

Vince shined his flashlight at the flying apparition. *What was it?*

It wasn't more that eighteen inches tall, had a lavender body, except for its tummy which was orange. It had black wings on its back which were rapidly beating against the air. Its eyes glowed red, illuminated by the flashlight. There were long sharp claws on its feet and shorter claws on its hands. Its mouth was closed, but there were sharp teeth pointing upwards.

"A dragon?" Vince and I both concluded, almost in unison.

"Daddy, daddy," the little dragon cried out, staring at Vince.

"It thinks I'm its Daddy," Vince whispered as we both crouched behind some boxes on the floor.

"If you're its daddy, then go to take care of it, give it a spanking or something," I hissed between my clenched teeth.

"You're the doctor," he responded. "Don't you think you should check it out, you know, just to be sure it's not injured or something?"

At this moment the lights came on and Maggie came in.

I jumped up and grabbed her as fire shot towards the door. Vince jumped up and raced towards the little monster.

"Aieee..." screamed the little dragon and then it flew into Vince's arms.

"Daddy, Daddy," it screamed again. And then, much to everyone's surprise, it licked Vince's face and threw its short arms around his neck.

Maggie and I slowly stood up, wary of the baby dragon's intentions, but Vince showed no fear as he looked up at us, the little beast still clutching his neck.

"I guess he's adopted you, Vince," I observed.

"I guess so," he answered. "Poor little guy. I bet he's all alone in the world; last of his kind no doubt."

"No doubt," I agreed.

Vince put the dragon down and held its hand. They made an odd looking couple. Tall elderly man and short squat monster.

"You know, Doc, I've been alone for years now. Lizzy's been gone for a long time and the kids are all grown and moved away. I was never big on pets, but I think I can make an exception."

"Just be careful, you don't want to end up half broiled," I remarked as the three of us walked back towards the break room.

"What do dragons eat?" Maggie asked.

"No idea," I stated. "He's sort of lizard like. Maybe insects or fish?"

"Maybe he's a vegetarian," Vince suggested.

Maggie sat down and took out a cigarette. As she put it to her lips a short flame shot out from the dragon and lit it. The flame, just reaching the end of the cigarette, carefully measured not to scorch anything else.

"Well, you'll need to give it a name. Is it a boy or a girl?" Maggie asked.

"Good question," Vince replied. He eyed his new charge up and down from every angle.

"What do you think, Doc?"

"No idea. Maybe we can do some DNA testing."

"What about Pat or Robin or Courtney?" Maggie suggested. "Those are all good names for either boys or girls."

"Daddy, daddy," the dragon cried out. "I'm hungry."

Maggie opened the refrigerator door and said, "Help yourself."

The little dragon half walked and half flew over to the fridge and grabbed my sandwich off the shelf and wolfed it down. Then it ate an apple, two oranges (which had belonged to Maggie), and drank a carton of milk.

"From what I can see," I remarked, "food is not going to be an issue."

I looked at my watch. "It's almost seven. I think you should be on your way with your adopted monster, Vince. The less explaining we have to do, the better."

He agreed. He dressed the dragon in a gray hoodie which we kept around for just such emergencies and left, holding his new pet's hand. As he walked away I called out:

"What are you going to call him or her?"

He screamed back an answer, but I couldn't quite make it out. At that moment Maggie handed me my coat. It was quitting time. Another eventful Night Clinic had come to an end.

Night Clinic and the Seven Dwarfs

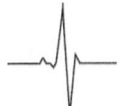

"I'M BACK," I ANNOUNCED AS I WALKED THROUGH THE back door to the clinic. "Did you miss me?"

I hadn't worked a shift at the Night Clinic for two months. A required rotation through the ICU had me on call every other night. Miss James turned and walked away, silently.

What did I do to her?

I couldn't keep from staring as I watched those shapely legs and derriere disappear into the supply room.

She emerged a few seconds later and gave me a big smile.

"Of course I've missed you," she finally answered. "No monsters or superheroes or dragons for months."

"So, you heard about my last little adventure, a bit scary at least for a few moments. Maybe tonight will be different. I say we should have a nice boring shift. Nothing but sick babies, winos, hookers with STD's, stabbings, gunshots, and drug overdoses for a change."

"You're cute," she remarked, patting my cheek. "Speaking of winos, there's one waiting for you in Exam 3, Alvin, a regular: diabetic, congestive heart failure, obese, drinks about a quart a day. Says he's short of breath."

I gave her my best Groucho Marx leer and picked up the chart on the door. Alvin was fifty-five years old, had a list of medications a mile long and usually was seen at the University Clinic. His vital signs were HR 80, BP 210/90, RR 28, O2 sat 88%. I took a deep breath and went in to see him.

"Hello, Mr. Gates, I'm Dr. Barnes," I introduced myself, smiling, and held out my hand to shake his. He was sitting on the edge of the exam table staring at the floor. His lips were a slightly blue and he was taking short rapid breaths.

"I'm sorry, Dr. Barnes. I mean for not getting up. I can't seem to catch my breath."

"When did you notice you were having difficulty?" Alvin was very large, his weight on the chart was listed as 350 pounds, but I would have guessed he was at least 450. He was dressed in a sleeveless t-shirt and dirty khaki pants, the tops of which were hidden by his massive belly. The t-shirt was drenched in sweat. He had worn out sandals on his feet, one of the straps replaced by some rough twine. The smell of dried sweat and spoiled wine filled the room.

"I never breathe real good, but it was last night. I guess I forgot to take my meds."

"Forgot for how long?" I asked as I fastened an oxygen mask around his head, which was in addition to the nasal cannula he already sported. The pulse oximeter fell to 84 while he was talking, but rose to 89 with the additional oxygen.

"I guess I missed going to the clinic last week and then I ran out of some of my medicines, but I just took double the dose of some of the others; I figured it would be OK. I guess I was wrong."

"Can you tell me what you did take?"

"Let's see. I took four of the big blue ones, no five, and one of the little white pills, three green capsules. I used the big inhaler and the small one two times yesterday and two times today. Took my water pill…"

Alvin's voice trailed off as he turned a darker shade of blue.

"Alvin… ALVIN," I shouted as I stood up and shook him.

"Wha… oh, sorry, Dr. Barnes. Sometimes I sort of pass out for a few seconds. Where was I? Oh, yeah, pills."

"Never mind, Alvin. I think you need to be at the hospital. We'll call an ambulance."

I left the room and asked Miss James to call the University ambulance crew. I started an IV on poor Alvin, drew some basic labs and Miss James did an EKG. Alvin's lungs crackled everywhere and his feet and ankles were giant tree trunks of brownish edema, but, surprisingly, no ulcers.

I gave him 80 of Lasix and waited for the ambulance.

While Miss James sat with him, I treated a two-year-old with an earache, a drug addict with an infected arm, splinted a sprained ankle and broken finger. When the ambulance finally arrived, I helped load Alvin onto the stretcher and wished him well as he rolled out the door.

I was looking forward to a few moments of quiet when I heard a loud thud outside the clinic door and a car's squealing tires as it raced away. Miss James and I investigated the noise and found a young woman, a young and very attractive woman, passed out on our doorstep. Her beauty would have rivaled Helen of Troy with long black hair, soft white skin, and bright red lips. She was dressed in a royal blue dress which clung to her every curve and had dark blue boots which came up to her knees. There was a ring on her left hand with a large blue stone which sparkled in the waiting room light.

We managed to get her into Exam Room 1. All the while she didn't move, didn't open her eyes, didn't even moan. She just lay like a rag doll on my exam table. She had no ID, no purse, no place to hide any money.

"If she's a working girl, she's done a good job of hiding her earnings," I commented.

"Probably robbed, hit over the head, and dumped here," Miss James concluded.

I listened to her heart which was clear and regular, her pulse was strong, lips, fingers, toes all pink, her respirations were regular. Pulse oximeter read 99%.

"She looks quite serene lying there on the table, almost like she's been enchanted," Miss James observed.

Her words were prescient as a loud noise, followed by shouting, came from the waiting room. I ran out to see about all the commotion and found seven "little" people at the reception desk, one was banging on the bell and another was pounding his walking stick on the desk.

"May I help you, Mr..." I asked. The dwarf was about three feet tall, with a large red nose and a long gray beard. He was dressed in a black suit and had a gold ring in his left ear.

"Where is she?" he demanded banging his stick on the reception desk. "Where is Crystal Blue?"

"And you are...?"

"Sleazy, if you must know. And behind me are Slutty, Skanky, Busty, Hunky, Tiny, and Norman."

"Seven dwarfs, huh?" I observed. "I would have thought you would have been named Happy, Sneezy, Bashful, Dopey, Grumpy, Sleepy, and Doc."

"We prefer 'little people' and those would be silly names for us. But, back to the matter at hand. Where is Crystal Blue? She works for me and I expect her out on that stage in ten minutes."

Miss James appeared and exclaimed, "You're from that place over on 14th, the "Enchanted Room."

"If you please, Nurse, it's 'The Enchanted Emporium Club' a place where men and women can leave all their worries and cares behind," Sleazy explained. "Now getting back to Crystal..."

"One moment, please," Miss James said and then motioned for me to follow her.

"Legally, we can't let these little people do anything or even see Crystal Blue, assuming that is her name. Maybe, we should call the police."

"Perhaps," I answered, "but no one has broken any laws and our first responsibility is to our comatose patient. The dwarfs will have to wait."

I went back to the reception desk and spoke to Sleazy.

"Crystal Blue, if that is her name, is sick. She seems to be asleep and won't wake up. I certainly cannot release her to just anyone and she is in no condition to perform. You and your companions are welcome to wait for her here in the waiting room."

I left them and went back to attend to my patient. By this time some of the tests were available.

"Let's see," I mumbled. "CBC is normal, chemistry normal, pregnancy test negative, UA negative, tox screen negative. Chest X-Ray... whoa, what's that?"

I stared at the film. The lungs were clear, but the cardiac silhouette was more than unusual. It looked like an apple; not just a vague apple-like appearance. It looked like someone had taken the outline of a perfect apple and pasted it where her heart was supposed to be.

Some new tropical disease? Apple fever? Apple poisoning? Maybe I should begin looking for the evil queen. As these thoughts popped into my head, Miss James appeared.

"A new patient has just arrived, Dr. Barnes," she announced.

"Nothing too serious I hope, Miss James. I'm sort of in a quandary with Miss Blue."

"I think you are going to want to see her right away. She's been beaten up pretty badly."

"OK, OK, I'll be right there."

I took a quick look at Crystal Blue before I left. She lay on the table quietly breathing, her chest silently heaving up and down.

I guess she's OK.

My new patient was in the exam room next door. Miss James was hard at work removing her tight fitting, sequined body suit. There were bruises on her face and arms and as the suit slowly came off there was a bruising and abrasions across her chest, abdomen, and pelvis.

"Do we have a name, Miss James."

"You won't believe this, but this is the Wicked Queen. At least that's her stage name. Her real name is Margaret Henson."

"Don't tell me. She works at the Enchanted Emporium Club as a dancer."

I gave her a quick exam. Her vital signs were normal, she was breathing normally and, although groggy, she was able to answer questions.

"Ms. Henson, I'm Dr. Barnes. Can you tell me what happened?"

"Wha... what happened?" she asked as she gradually became more alert. She started to sit up, but winced and then lay back down.

"It looks like you've been roughed up pretty badly. What hurts the most?"

"My chest, every time I try to breathe."

I'd already put oxygen on her and Miss James had an IV running in her left arm.

"Any abdominal pain?" I began taking a more thorough history.

"No, just my chest, on the right side."

I pulled up her spandex top and saw bruising all across her chest and upper abdomen.

"Do you have any medical problems, take any medicine regularly, any allergies?" I asked.

"No, no, and no. I don't smoke, drink alcohol, or use any type of illicit drugs. My only vice is that I take off my clothes to entertain degenerate men and once in a while leave with one, if he is cute enough and rich enough."

She finished her speech and then winced as she took a deep breath.

"Well, Ms. Henson. If I were a betting man, I would wager that you have some fractured ribs on the right side. We'll get a chest x-ray just to be sure. Can you tell me what happened?"

"I was ambushed. Somebody snuck up behind me and 'WHAM' on the back of my head, then 'WHACK' across my chest. Next thing I know this cute doctor is standing over me poking and prodding and feeling all my unmentionable parts."

"It's my job, Ms. Henson, figuring out what's wrong and then trying to fix it. Now if you will sit in this chair, Miss James will wheel you down the hall for an x-ray. In the mean time, I will have a little chat with the seven dwarfs."

Miss James wheeled her away, asking her what it was like to take off her clothes in front of a bunch of strangers. I couldn't hear the answer as they disappeared into the x-ray suite. I went up to the reception area.

"Sleazy, could you come back here, now," I commanded.

All seven little people followed him into Exam Room Three.

I turned and addressed Sleazy.

"Miss Henson accuses you of assaulting her. Is she correct in her assessment? Before you say too much, I must inform you that I am obligated to report the incident to the police."

"Miss Henson, the Wicked Queen, you mean, or the Wicked Witch, as we like to call her, works for me and is never happy. I'm sure she cannot name the name of her assailant as it is obvious from her injuries that she was attacked from behind. I would also like to add that it is almost certain that this Wicked Queen poisoned Crystal Blue and she will most definitely try to bump her off again if she is allowed the opportunity. That witch hates our poor Crystal."

The other six dwarfs echoed Sleazy's sentiments.

"Why," I inquired, "this severe animosity between Ms. Henson and Ms. Blue?"

Sleazy sat down in the lone chair, stroked his gray beard and began his story. His six companions sat on the floor as the story commenced.

"I opened the Enchanted Emporium about two years ago. My original intent was to create a place where the outcasts of society could congregate without feeling self conscious. The seven of us manage the club. We started just with a bar and a bunch of large TV screens and video games, like every other bar and club. It was Norman who hit on the idea of adding the live entertainment. So, we hired a few girls of various size and shape. It wasn't long before I learned that there are a lot of people willing to take off their clothes for money and a lot of people who will pay to see it. And, this is where we really stand out from the crowd, because it isn't just the mainstream 'beautiful' girl who can find an audience. Fat, thin, tall, short, young, old, every size and shape, male or female has an audience somewhere. Surely, you've heard of our geriatric night? No?

Well, it always draws them in. But I'm getting off the track.

"The Wicked Queen started working about eighteen months ago and she was a big hit. She's beautiful in the traditional sense, all the attributes that make for a successful dancer, big shapely chest, cute butt, and she did magic. While she performed, she made snakes appear and change into birds, turned cats into dogs, and other such tricks. There was the time she made a particularly unruly patron disappear; I don't think he was ever found.

"Anyway, she ruled the runway for more than a year. Until Crystal showed up. Crystal Blue, that's even her real name, came from somewhere in the Midwest. She just got on the bus and ended up here, running away or going somewhere, I don't know and she has never told us. I think she was one of the lost souls living on the streets for a while who happened to wander into our little club one night.

"Even through her ragged clothes I could tell she was a real beauty with an air about her that made her special. I'm not sure if it was her innocence or quiet charm, or what. I do know that I and my fellow managers were captivated from the start. She worked as a barmaid at first, but then asked if she could try her hand at performing. She certainly had the look and she could sing, too.

"She didn't have the typical exotic dancer body; only medium boobs, but very shapely tush, and she radiates charm, and she has such a sweet voice. She was a big hit from the start. Every time she was out on that stage it was magical. Well, you can imagine the trouble, the jealousy, the envy. I'm not surprised it came to this."

At this moment, Miss James interrupted.

"Here's the chest x-ray on the Wicked Queen, Dr. Barnes," she reported.

"Excuse me, fellas, but I need to check this."

As I suspected, the Queen had fractured ribs four through ten on the right side with maybe a contusion to the lung. There was no pneumothorax or effusion. I went and checked on my two patients before hearing the rest of the story. Crystal Blue continued in her serene and unrelenting sleep, while the Queen was sitting up in the chair and appeared to be fairly comfortable. I informed her of the x-ray results, listened to her chest again, checked her vital signs and abdomen. I asked her to wait a bit longer so that I could evaluate her one more time before she left, but I also hoped I could get some information on what had happened to the comatose Ms. Blue.

I left and returned to hear more of Sleazy's story.

"Tell him about the mirror," one of the other dwarfs, Slutty, I think, interjected.

"Don't tell me she has a magic mirror on the wall, as in 'Mirror, Mirror on the wall who's the sleaziest of them all?' " I said.

"No, no, nothing like that, at least I don't think so. She, does, however, stand in front of the mirror for long periods of time, hours it seems, primping her hair, talking to herself. It's a bit bizarre if you ask me. Old Mamba says it's all just vanity."

"Who's Old Mamba?" I just had to ask.

"She's our cleaning lady, a withered old prune from Haiti. I think she's about a million years old," Tiny explained, in a high squeaky voice. "But, she and the Wicked Queen have some sort of thing going on, because they're always together."

"Tell me, Sleazy," I asked, "what happened to your star dancer tonight? Did Crystal Blue suffer some sort of psychotic breakdown leaving her in a catatonic state? Or, did the Wicked Queen trick her into eating a poisoned apple which plunged her into an everlasting sleep only to be awakened by true love's kiss? Or is it something else?"

Miss James stuck her head in the room at that moment.

"Chest pain in Four; an old black lady, looks like it might be bad."

"On my way, Nurse," I replied. "We'll pick this up in a few minutes, lads." I left the little people and went to attend to my patient. For some reason, Norman followed me.

"That's Old Mamba," he cried out and all the other dwarfs suddenly appeared.

"You all need to wait outside," I said sternly and Miss James ushered them out.

I glanced at the monitor and saw very elevated ST segments on her EKG with an irregular rhythm with frequent PVC's and a BP that was 80/50.

"This does not look good, Nurse. Mamba, can you hear me?"

My question was answered by a long groan. Miss James was on the phone calling for an ambulance as I started an IV, put oxygen on Old Mamba, and started a Lidocaine infusion along with low dose Dopamine. Her oxygen saturation was around 90 even with O2. Her lungs had crackles from top to bottom.

"Get the crash cart," I mumbled, but Miss James was ahead of me.

"V fib," I shouted. I intubated the old woman as Miss James started CPR and warmed up the paddles to shock the dying woman.

Epi, bicarb, bag, shock, compress, repeat, nothing worked. I even brought the dwarfs in to help with chest compressions, but we lost her.

After thirty minutes the ambulance arrived and was sent away. Miss James went through the layers of poor Old Mamba's clothing, which lay in a heap on the floor.

"What's this?" she muttered as she folded the dress.

Madame Marie's Incantations and Spells: The Complete Guide to Withcraft and Voodoo by Marie, Voodoo High Priestess.

"And, what's this?" Miss James pulled out a likeness of Crystal Blue.

"Perhaps it was Old Mamba who put a spell on poor Crystal," Busty remarked.

Miss James was thumbing through the book.

"Dr. Barnes," she shouted out suddenly. "This particular spell is circled. It's called the 'Living Death'."

"Let me look at that, please," I requested.

"Voodoo doll... lock of hair... two dead chickens... incantation and douse with... Miss James, did you notice the funny smell in Room One?"

"Come to think of it, I did, sort of like cinnamon mixed with fruit."

"That's right, cinnamon and apples. It looks like Old Mamba cast this spell on poor Miss Blue. I suspect our other patient, the Queen, may be able to tell us more."

At this moment we all heard a scream from Exam Room Two. All of us raced into the room and found Norman standing on the exam table with a scalpel held to the throat of the Wicked Queen.

"Admit it," he screamed with an almost comical high-pitched voice. "Tell everyone how you cursed poor Crystal Blue. Say it or you'll be joining Old Mamba."

Skanky tried to calm his companion. "Now, Norman, I know you have no great love for the Wicked Queen, but are sure about her? I ask because the doctor and nurse found this in Old Mamba's clothes."

He held up the voodoo doll and book. Norman only squinted and then held the knife tighter to the Wicked Queen's throat so that drops of blood started to well up.

Busty stepped in and started to approach Norman.

"Norman, Norman, I know you're upset about our dear Crystal Blue. She's always been so sweet and loving. Even if the Queen did cast a spell, do we want to stoop down to her level?"

Busty's voice was even higher than Norman's. She (or was it he) had smooth skin, except for a bit of stubble on the chin and a big chest, but her manner was very masculine.

"Busty used to be Brutus, before all the treatment and surgery," Slutty whispered to me. Busty kept right on walking towards Norman. Norman started to hold the knife even tighter against the Queen's throat as blood started to run down her neck. Busty stopped and Norman relaxed for a moment.

"Ow," Norman squeaked.

Miss James grabbed his arm as she pulled the needle from his buttock and the Wicked Queen broke free from Norman's hold. Norman slowly slumped to the ground as I ran to examine the Queen's wounds, then held a wad of sterile gauze against the laceration to stop the bleeding. She broke away from me and delivered a sharp kick to Norman's side.

I finally reached the point where I just couldn't take it any more.

I yelled at the top of my lungs, "EVERYONE STOP, JUST STOP, RIGHT NOW!" I let my voice drop a few decibels as Miss James joined me at my side.

"Now, listen, all of you. There will be no more knives or spells or anything. Everyone out to the waiting room and sit. Not you, Ms. Henson, not until I can check your neck more closely to see if you need any stitches. Miss James, would you please call the police and the coroner for Old Mamba. Thank you."

The seven dwarfs slowly made their way out to the waiting room. Sleazy started to speak, but I held up my finger gesturing for him to be silent. I examined the Queen's neck more closely. The cut was superficial and had stopped bleeding. I cleaned it with Betadine, then dried it, steri-stripped it closed, and applied a new, sterile dressing. I then motioned for her and Miss James to follow me out to the waiting room.

The Queen sat alongside the seven dwarfs, while Miss James stood by me. I stared out at a bizarre scene, the wicked Queen dressed in black Spandex, seven "little" people sporting beards, dressed in outfits ranging from seventies leisure suits to Sleazy's black suit and red bowtie. I paused for a moment before I spoke. Sleazy tried to speak, but I signaled that he should be silent.

"You have made this one of the more unusual night's we've experienced here at the Clinic," I began, "and that is quite a trick considering some of the bizarre things that manage to pass through those doors. But, we have had assaults, magical spells, and death join us here, and it is now time to get to the bottom of this. I will start with you, Ms. Henson. Do you have knowledge regarding the illness which has come upon Crystal Blue?"

At first the Queen just sat there.

"I promise you, Ms. Henson, that if you are truthful your diminutive employers will do you no more harm. Isn't that so, Mr. Sleazy?"

I waited for a reply and then repeated, a bit more forcefully, "I said, isn't that so, Mr. Sleazy?"

"Yeah..." he answered, barely audible.

"What?" I responded.

"Yes, we won't hurt her anymore," Sleazy answered, clearly. His six companions nodded in agreement.

"Now, Ms. Henson, what do you know about voodoo and witchcraft, as practiced by the now deceased Old Mamba?"

The Queen looked around and seemed a bit embarrassed, but finally spoke.

"I did mention, one time to Old Mamba, that I wished Crystal Blue was gone. That I had been the top girl until she showed up. But, that's all. I never asked her to do anything. Well, maybe she saw me moping about and she would ask me what was wrong and I'd point to something blue or make some sort of gesture. I never thought she would or even could cast such a spell."

"But, you are always doing magic as part of your act," Sleazy observed.

"Sure, cheap parlor tricks I learned from an old boyfriend, pull some flowers from a hat or make a bird disappear. You never saw me do anything else, did you?" the Queen asked, her question directed to everyone listening.

There was a general murmuring that actually did agree with her.

"It seems, however, that Old Mamba has managed to cast a true spell, or drug or hypnotize or something to Ms. Blue; there is no question," I observed. "Living Death. That's the spell she circled in her voodoo book. Do any of you know anything about it; how to break the spell?"

"In the old story, it was true love's kiss what worked," one of the dwarfs, Hunky, I think, remarked.

"Well, that may be as good a place to start as any," I decided. I, for one, was stumped. Narcan didn't do anything; allowing time for a drug to metabolize wasn't accomplishing anything. There was no mark on Crystal that would suggest she was injected with anything. Her liver, renal, and respiratory function were all normal. She just wouldn't wake up. She did not respond to any neurologic stimulus, no posturing, no localizing of pain, no eye opening, nothing. And she looked peaceful, so peaceful sleeping, just sleeping. We didn't have a CT Scanner at the clinic, but I had no doubt it would have been normal. I turned back to the dwarfs.

"True love's kiss is as good a place as any to start," I announced. "Do any of you know if she has a boyfriend of any family?"

"She lives alone," Norman reported. "And, she's never mentioned any family. She used to say that our little emporium was her family. I guess it's kind of sad."

"Norman, don't you have a key to her apartment? Didn't she give you one in case there was some sort of emergency? This certainly qualifies as one," Sleazy said.

"Yup, got it right here," and he held up a key ring with about a hundred keys on it.

"What's with all the keys?" I had to ask.

"Well, let's see. This one is to my apartment, this one is to the Emporium, this one is to my mom's house, the front door and this other is to her back door. This one goes to my locker and …"

"Never mind, I get the picture. Now go see what you can find and take someone with you."

Skanky shot up his hand. "I'll go."

"OK, OK, check it out and bring back anything that will give us a clue as to the lovers in her life. Oh and before you leave, why don't you each give her a kiss; just in case one of you is her true love."

They looked at each other with a smirk on their faces and then rushed into Room One.

"Just on the cheek, you two, and just a light kiss."

They looked disappointed as they each planted a light kiss on her cheek. Nothing happened. They left to check out her apartment.

Each dwarf in turn planted a kiss on her cheek and even the Wicked Queen kissed her, all without success.

"What we really need is a handsome prince," I remarked. For completeness sake, Miss James and I also kissed her, with, thankfully, no results. Once all this kissing was finished, a police car pulled up.

Officers Kreplock and Jenson came in.

"Hey, Doc. Good evening, Miss James. What's going on?"

I proceeded to recount the events of the night with embellishments thrown in by Sleazy and Busty.

"So let me see if I've got this straight," Officer Kreplock summed up when we'd finished our story. "There has been some sort of assault on a stripper named Crystal Blue and two assaults on stripper Margaret Henson aka the Wicked Queen, the old cleaning lady from the strip joint may have been one perpetrator, but she's dead, while one or all of these seven dwarfs may also be perpetrators. Meanwhile two of these dwarfs are off on some sort of home investigation trying to find some clues as to the identity of the 'true love' of the now drugged or comatose Crystal Blue because you all have a wild idea that 'true love's kiss' will break the spell she's under and wake her up from her coma?"

"That's it in a nutshell, Officer," I replied.

"Doc, you've been watching too many late night movies. Let me call the hospital and get an ambulance over here to take your comatose patient to the hospital."

I looked him in the eye and then looked through the open door into exam room one and the peacefully sleeping Crystal Blue. I knew he was right to take her to the hospital. Still, I'd seen so many peculiar, bizarre occurrences, met innumerable weird and wonderful and eccentric patients here at the clinic that a magic spell cast over one of my patients just didn't strike me as being much out of the ordinary, at least for *this* Night Clinic.

"I'll tell you what, Officers," I negotiated, "just wait to see what the two dwarfs, Norman and Skanky discover. If we can't wake Miss Blue up, then we'll send her to the hospital."

"OK, Doc, as long as it's not too long a wait."

"Oh, it shouldn't be long. Here they are now. What did you find?"

Norman walked in empty handed.

"Well, her apartment is pretty empty. Nothing on the walls, no photos, no computer, no diary, no letters, nothing. But, while we were looking around we heard growling from the bathroom and found him."

Norman pointed outside where Skanky was wrestling with a big headstrong German Shepherd.

"At first he growled at us and bared his teeth as we searched around. But, I think he figured out we were there to help, because he calmed down after a few minutes. As we were leaving, feeling pretty much like failures he ran to the door with his leash in his mouth. I didn't think we had time to take him for a walk, but he wouldn't let us out the door unless we brought him along. I think he decided we would take him to see our poor Crystal."

"Keep him in the waiting room for now, please," I suggested, but then I thought for a moment. "No, wait, let him free."

Skanky and Norman looked confused, but then released the dog. The beast started barking and then bounded into Exam Room One and stood up on his hind legs and started licking Crystal Blue's face. As he did this, there started to be flashing lights of red and blue, a wind blew from nowhere, and a white light engulfed the dog and Miss Blue. We all stood by, dumbfounded, as the light and wind grew brighter and stronger and then suddenly stopped.

I half expected to find the room empty, while also half expecting Crystal Blue to walk out with a handsome prince on her arm. And, she did walk out, only with her dog at her side. The dog was not an enchanted prince. He was just a German Shepherd. He did have a tag, however, with his name engraved upon it. In big white letters it said: "PRINCE."

After this everyone filed out of the Clinic. News of the miraculous occurrences made the Enchanted Emporium a top tourist attraction and the popularity caused Sleazy to tone down some of the more unusual performances. Miss Henson and Miss Blue became fast friends and started an act together, playing to packed houses up and down the coast. Prince was prominently featured in the show.

After everyone had left it was just about quitting time. Miss James and I had breakfast together.

"I guess there's no love like a dog's love for its master. Prince sure proved that," Miss James sighed.

"Well, that is one kind of love and I certainly believe it is true love. Maybe you and I can discover some other type of love…"

Her eyes widened and then she stared down at her bacon.

"Why Dr. Barnes…" and she laughed as we finished our breakfast.

Night Clinic and the Garden

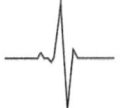

"DR. BARNES, HOW NICE TO SEE YOU AGAIN, IT'S BEEN TOO long," Miss James remarked as I hung up my coat. "Residency been busy?"

"You have no idea, Nurse. I wish people would only get sick between the hours of 8:30 and 5:00. It's so inconvenient when someone decides to have an MI at midnight. Personally, I wish my only night work was here at the Night Clinic."

I leaned over to give her a kiss, but she turned her head away. I guess two months was too long a time to let pass without seeing or calling her. *This could be a long shift,* I thought, but one never knows what may transpire to bring people back together.

"Anyone waiting?" I inquired, hoping I could break down her icy veneer.

"High fever and a rash in Two and vomiting in Three. Room One needs to be cleaned. It seems the day shift never went to kindergarten and left one a bit of a disaster."

I picked up the chart outside Room Two. Owen Martin, thirty-two, no previous medical problems, fever for three days, up to 103, and generalized rash. *Here we go.*

"Good evening, Mr. Martin, what brings you in here today?" I started my doctor banter.

"Bus," he answered tersely.

It's going to be one of those nights.

"I'm sorry," I started over. "I mean, what's the problem you're having."

"What's the problem, Doctor? Just look at me; you can see the problem."

"That is quite a rash, no question. When did it start and where did you first notice it?"

"I first noticed it in the bathroom about a week ago."

I raised an eyebrow at his response and then rephrased my question. "Where on your body did you first notice the rash?"

"Oh, sorry, Doctor. It was on my stomach. It just spread each day and then I noticed the fever and some aching in my joints."

"Been hiking in the woods recently; any bug bites?"

"I was hunting a couple of weeks ago. Didn't manage to kill anything, though, except about a case of beer."

Lyme disease popped into my head. "Did you get bitten by a tick? Let me check you. Go ahead and get undressed, here's a gown for you. I'll be back in a few minutes."

I left Mr. Martin and went to Room Three. Sixty years old... hypertension... vomiting today, nothing much. Probably a stomach bug. I noticed Miss James looking a bit frazzled as I opened the door.

"It's going to be a busy night. There are about ten people in the waiting room already."

I better pick it up.

"Good evening, Mr. Sanchez, what is the problem..."

I quickly dispatched him with a script for phenergan and follow up at the County Clinic in a few days and then went back to search for a tick.

"I'm back," I announced as I returned to Room Two. You said the rash started on your stomach?"

That's right, Doctor," Mr. Martin answered.

I started my search on his abdomen without any luck, moved to his groin and perineum, up and down, everywhere, but the nasty bug eluded me and my magnifying glass.

"What are you looking for, Doctor?" my patient queried.

"A bug, a tick to be exact."

"Oh," he answered and then he became quiet. After another

minute he spoke up. "I did find a little spider, maybe it was a tick, in my belly button. I killed it."

"Let me look at your belly button," I requested.

I pulled the skin apart to open it up and got up close and magnified the area. There was a tiny black speck that I pulled out. *This could be part of a tick.* I didn't see anything else.

"Mr. Martin, I suspect you have Lyme disease. Here is a prescription for antibiotics, one pill twice a day. It shouldn't be very expensive. Take it to the pharmacy over on Sixteenth. It should only be four dollars. Here is a sample to get you started. And, this is the number for the Infectious Disease Clinic at the hospital. See them within the next week or so. Don't forget to take the antibiotics and, here's another script for your aching and itching. Any questions?"

"I'm not going to die, am I, Dr. Barnes? I always heard about Lyme disease and…"

"We caught it early, Owen. Just take the medication and keep your appointment and you should be fine."

He shook my hand, clutching the prescriptions tightly in his other fist.

"Thanks, Dr. Barnes. I'll call you if I don't get better."

"Go to the Clinic if you don't get better, but be sure to go."

He left and I went out into the hall. All the rooms had charts on the door and I peeked out into the waiting room and saw about twenty more people seated. No one looked terribly ill until I saw her. She was a little girl sitting by herself in the corner, next to a fake potted plant. She sat with her hands across her knees, fidgeting.

Miss James came out of Exam Room One.

"Nurse," I formally requested, "there's a little girl sitting by herself in the corner out there. Please bring her back next. Thank you."

"Of course, Dr. Barnes."

I picked up the chart to Room Four. "Splinter in hand."

I opened the door and greeted Mr. Billroth. "Good evening, Mr…"

I went through my usual spiel, but my thoughts kept drifting back to that little girl. Something about her demeanor was unsettling. I quickly removed the splinter from Mr. Billroth and sent him on his way. I ignored the patients who had been waiting in Rooms One and Two and went to Three and the little girl.

Her chart was blank, no name, age, or anything.

"Hello," I said gently. "I'm Dr. Barnes. Can you tell me your name?"

She looked at me with her big brown eyes, but just sat there, clutching a raggedy doll to her chest. She couldn't have been more than five years old. Long, curly brown hair fell around her shoulders and she was neatly dressed in a blue dress and pink tennis shoes. She didn't have any of the grime I'd come to expect on "street orphans" which made me think that she had a home somewhere and she was probably lost or had just run away.

"I promise no one will hurt you."

Miss James came in behind me.

"We just want to know who you are and where your parents are."

"Daddy's at the hospital. Mommy was there, but they took her away and now she's in the garden. I saw her there today and I wanted to be with her, but she told me I had to leave."

Miss James knelt beside the little girl.

"What's your name, honey?" she asked while she slowly stroked her hair. The girl didn't answer.

"Can you tell me your doll's name?" I asked. "I'm sure she's scared, too."

The girl held up the doll, which looked worn and dirty.

"This is Peaches. Mommy gave her to me before she got sick and had to go to the hospital."

"Can you tell me your name?" Miss James asked again. "If Peaches gets lost, I'll know who you are and be able to bring her to you."

"Jewel," she answered. "My name is Jewel and I'm five years old. Please, I want to go back to the garden and be with Mommy."

I took Miss James aside for a moment.

"Do you know of any garden near here? All I've ever seen is garbage and dirt and more garbage."

She shook her head and went back to Jewel.

"Can you tell me about the garden?" she asked.

"It was wonderful, so beautiful and smelled so sweet and fresh. I saw Mommy there. I wanted to go with her, but I couldn't."

"Where is the garden? I asked.

"It wasn't far from here. Mommy was at the hospital. She's had to go there a lot. I was there with Daddy, but then they took Mommy away. I couldn't stand it so I ran away to find her. And I did find her; in the garden."

"Can you tell me about the garden, Jewel?"

"There were beautiful flowers and birds and even a lion. There was a river which sparkled in the sun and Mommy was sitting in the middle of it and she didn't look sick at all. She looked happy and pretty and I wanted to go with her. I tried to run to her, but she told me I had to wait. 'Someday we would be together again,' she said. Then she went away again and then I couldn't find the garden anymore. But, I was standing right outside your door after Mommy left. Every other place looked dark and dirty, but it was light here, so I came inside. Please, can't you go with me to find the garden again?"

I looked at Jewel and then at Miss James, but didn't say anything. Finally, I told Jewel to wait in the exam room while Miss James and I talked about what to do.

"It's obvious what's happened. Her mother must have been sick and died at a hospital. When she learned that her mother had been taken away she ran away to find her and imagined her to be in a beautiful garden. Probably a pretty healthy defense mechanism for the little girl. I think that our task is to figure out which hospital her mother was in, which will help us find her father so we can get her home. Why don't you start calling the hospitals and I'll take care of the other patients."

"Sounds like a reasonable plan, Dr. Barnes. I'll keep Jewel with me," Miss James replied.

We went to separate ends of the clinic. Miss James was in the back office while I saw a stream of patients with, luckily, minor complaints. Headaches, backaches, foot aches, neck aches, sore throats, sore ears, sore eyes, they all came and went. It was four a.m. when I finally had the clinic cleared out and I could check on Jewel and Miss James.

"Any luck?" I asked.

Jewel was sitting on the floor drawing, while Miss James was scribbling something on the pad.

"Mercy Hospital, Saucedo, you'll contact her father. OK, but can you give me his contact information, thanks," she finished her phone conversation and turned towards me. "Her name is Jewel Saucedo, she just turned five years old and her mother, Mary, just passed away. She had been battling ovarian cancer for a couple of years."

"Do we know where the father is?"

"His cell phone is 906-100-1000. They called him while I was on the phone with them and he's on his way here."

"Good, good. At least I managed to clear out all those patients. I'm glad none of them were terribly sick," I commented, then I turned towards Jewel. "Jewel, your dad is on his way... Jewel... JEW-EL."

I was shouting because our little Jewel was gone. We called everywhere in the clinic, but she didn't answer. Only her drawing remained, a picture of green trees, colorful birds, and a woman with long dark hair. Jewel's Garden. I was starting to feel a bit frantic, first because a little girl was out alone in the night in what could be a dangerous part of town and second because her father was on his way and expecting to find his little girl safe at the Clinic.

"Call the police and her father and tell them what's going on. Close the Clinic for the rest of the night. I'm going out to find her. You wait here in case she comes back."

I raced out into the night, shouting her name, "JEWEL, JEW-EL."

I went from street to street. I saw police cars roll by several times and stopped and talked to two of the officers. No luck so far.

If anything should happen to her…

But I couldn't think anymore about that.

It was beginning to get lighter as I was becoming more discouraged. But, then I saw something unusual, extraordinary, wonderful. At first I thought it was the sunrise, but it was to the west and was too bright. A light shining in the distance. I ran towards it and when I saw it I froze.

There, across the wide boulevard, was Jewel's garden. In the middle of dark gray buildings, piles of unclaimed garbage, rats, winos, and urban blight was the most beautiful garden I had ever seen. Lush green trees and plants, vibrant, bright flowers, birds with feathers of every color singing and calling; the most splendid beauty filled my eyes. I heard the rush of a swift river and then I saw them, sitting on the far side of the river, mother and daughter, Mary and Jewel, laughing together, happy, more than happy, joyful.

I started to cross the wide street and Jewel looked up at me and waved. As I stepped out in the street I heard the shrill wail of a car horn and stepped back as an eighteen-wheeler rolled past. When I looked up, Mary, Jewel and the garden were gone. All that remained was Jewel's worn, torn doll. I picked it up and trudged slowly across the street.

I knew I would never find them again, but I also knew that little Jewel was where she belonged. I started to walk back to the clinic, slowly at first, but then I began to run. I was out of breath when I finally made it back, barely noticing the flashing lights as I went inside.

"MISS JAMES. MISS JAMES," I shouted as I walked past the waiting room.

"I'm here," she answered softly. Her eyes were filled with tears.

Before she could speak, I blurted out, "I saw, her, Jewel, and her mother. And Jewel's garden. And they were so happy, so peaceful..."

"SHE'S DEAD, JEWEL'S DEAD," and Miss James broke down crying.

I held my assistant tightly and stroked her hair, not knowing what to say or do. At the same time, her words didn't surprise me. I suppose I already knew the truth, but after seeing her and her mother and their garden, I couldn't feel sad. I left Miss James and went to speak to the police and a very distraught father.

"She was hit by a bus crossing Elm. Happened about an hour and half ago. The bus driver said he honked and tried to stop, but..."

"Is this her father?" I inquired. There was a man of about thirty, eyes bloodshot and sunken, weariness and anguish radiated from the center of his being.

"Leon Saucedo," he whispered.

"May I speak to you in private?" I requested. He nodded his head.

I took him into one of the exam rooms and told him my story. I hoped it would provide a tiny amount of solace. He thanked me and went away, carrying Jewel's ragged doll.

I filled in all the details for the police and they went away. Finally, we were alone. Only Miss James and I remained in the clinic. The next shift would be arriving in less than an hour. I went back to her and sat down on the floor next to her. She was crying, deep sobs and wails. I handed her a towel and then told her.

"You know, what Jewel told us about the garden was true. I saw it. It was all she said and more. It was like a glimpse into Heaven here on earth. And when you told me she was dead, I already knew it, but, I couldn't, can't, feel sad, after seeing her in that place. As a matter of fact, I wished I could be with them. More than anything I wanted to be with them. I started to cross the street, and I felt such joy, but I had to stop when a truck came by and then it was too late.

I suppose it wasn't my time, wasn't meant to be. I don't know if it's all good or bad, but I do know one thing. Among all the memorable and extraordinary days and nights I've lived as a doctor, in the hospital or here at the clinic, this is the most memorable and amazing of them all."

Her cries stopped and she stared at me.

"Dr. Barnes, I don't know what I would do without you. It's never boring with you around; you most definitely brighten up my mundane life."

She put her arm around me and gave me a light kiss on the cheek as we waited for our shift to end.

Beam Me Up Night Clinic

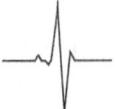

"OF COURSE *YOU'RE* WORKING TONIGHT," MISS JAMES stated. "Wherever and whenever there are bizarre events, that's where Dr. Barnes will be."

"I don't know what you mean, Nurse. It's been five weeks since my last shift here; are you telling me it's been nothing but chest pain, abdominal pain, and PIA?"

"Let's just say that I haven't seen a dragon in weeks."

Can I help if all the crazies come out when I'm working? It's not like I carry them with me.

"Speaking of bizarre and crazy, you are aware that the Intergalactic Convention is in town again? Star Trek, Star Wars, and every other outer space franchise all together. So I'm sure we'll get our share of phaser burns, blaster bruises, and transporter malfunctions. Oh, and to get us off on the right foot, Derek is back with his annual 'Trouble with Tribbles.' I've left all the usual instruments in the room for you."

"Not again," I moaned. "You would think that after four, no five years, he would learn."

I picked up the chart and gave it a careless glance. Before I saw the words I knew the problem. I walked into the exam room and saw Derek, a regular visitor, lying on his side on the exam table. Seated on a sterile tray were a rigid sigmoidoscope and a tenaculum.

"Derek, we've got to stop meeting like this," I scolded. "And think of the poor Tribbles. They're supposed to be comforting, I know, but you're just supposed to hold them."

"I do hold them, Dr. Barnes; for a little while. But, the way they coo and vibrate and shake, the possibilities are endless."

"I hope it's as simple as last year," I remarked.

I put on a glove and lubed up my index finger and checked up in Derek's rectum. Sure enough there was a furry object vibrating just inside. Past experience told me not to try to grab it with my hand; it would just slip away. I greased up the scope and passed it into his rectum. Immediately I visualized a furry yellow ball which was shaking and making low Tribble noises. I reached in with the tenaculum and grabbed the object in its mid portion like a pro and pulled scope and tenaculum out with a single, gentle pull. The Tribble, which was a toy available at the convention, popped out.

"Just one this year?" I asked, although I already knew there would be more.

"No, three," he replied.

I repeated the routine, pulling out one purple and one red Tribble, both larger that the first and still vibrating.

"I'll dispose of these for you, Derek. And, please, stay away from Tribbles. You know they're nothing but trouble."

He gave a short grunt as I walked out of the exam room.

"What's next, Nurse?"

"Intractable vomiting in Room One after imbibing 'Romulan Ale'; Darth Vader is in Two with a couple of storm troopers."

"Room One sounds easier," I commented as I picked up the chart outside the door.

"Kang... unusual name," I murmured to myself as I opened the door. "Good evening, Mr. Kang. I'm Dr. Barnes. What seems to be the problem?"

I was greeted by a dark-faced, sweaty man with a goatee, dressed in some sort of outer space uniform, seated on the chair, supporting a basin between his legs. As I approached him, he violently vomited into the basin, a dark, violet fluid.

"Curse this Romulan ale," he sneered. "You think I would have learned by now."

"When did this vomiting start?" I asked while feeling his pulse. His wrist was wet with perspiration and he felt warm. His heart was beating at about one twenty.

"With the first swig of that vile liquid. I should stick with our own Blood wine. Klingons make by far the most potent drink in the Universe."

"I'm sure you do, Mr. Kang."

"It's just Kang."

"Of course." I examined his eyes, looked down his throat, listened to his heart and lungs, palpated his abdomen, and then wrote him a prescription for Carafate and Phenergan, and sent him on his way. He didn't utter a word of gratitude.

On to Darth Vader.

I picked up the chart on the door. Shortness of breath, hoarseness… no age… no address. I knocked and opened the door to find myself staring at two Storm Troopers aiming what I assumed were fake blasters at me, while Lord Vader sat in the chair, head held high, his right fist clenched tightly. I raised my arms in mock surrender.

"Don't shoot, I'm only the doctor," I exclaimed. "Dr. Barnes, Lord Vader. What seems to be the problem?"

I heard the whoosh of jets from his black-armored suit and then a raspy, shallow breath.

"I seem to have trouble breathing," he answered, his voice deep but punctuated with a definite wheeze. "The Force is ebbing away from me."

"When did you start noticing the problem?" I inquired in my usual doctor tone.

"I've been pursuing rebel warriors from one end of the galaxy to the other. The Force had been strong with me, but since I've come to this place I've suffered."

"Hmm, it seems your Force has more sense than you; this is not the best part of town. However, I was referring to the breathing difficulty. Can you take that black outfit off so that I can examine you properly?"

"Dr. Barnes, I don't believe you completely comprehend my situation. My life and very being depend upon this suit. It is designed to maintain the power that flows to me from the Dark Side."

"Dark Side, Light Side, I don't know how I'm supposed to treat you if I can't properly examine you."

"I find your condescending attitude disturbing, Dr. Barnes."

"Listen, Mr. Vader. I know there's an 'Intergalactic Convention' here in town, but you're in my clinic now and you came to me for help, so give me a break, will you? I'm trying to help you. OK... OK, let me listen to your lungs through your armor."

I moved closer and pressed my stethoscope tightly against his back. He flinched a little. I was able to detect a definite expiratory wheeze and even a slight inspiratory wheeze bilaterally. His expiratory phase was markedly prolonged.

"Seems to be an asthma attack, Mr. Vader. A bit of a breathing treatment should fix you right up. Let me find the nurse and she will administer the medication. Where should she put it? It's designed to be inhaled."

He fumbled with his black suit and exposed an injection port. I noticed his light saber at his side.

"The medicine can go in here," he stated.

I left Lord Vader and his Storm Troopers, gave the orders to Miss James and went on to the next room.

Light Saber injury... Mr. Spock. Mixing space themes, this could be interesting.

I knocked on the door and went in holding my hand up in the Vulcan salute. "Live long and prosper, Mr. Spock; I've always wanted to say that and really mean it," I quipped.

Seated in the room was a dead ringer for Mr. Spock, a deep gash across his lower chest with exposed ribs and charred tissue dotted with greenish black stains, just what one would expect after being slashed with a light saber. Standing next to the injured party was a companion, Captain Kirk, I presumed.

"Mr. Spock had a run-in with a tall raspy villain, dressed in black armor. He was slashed with his weapon, some sort of laser sword. Patch him up, Doc. We have an appointment in two hours that we cannot miss." Kirk explained.

"One hour fifty four minutes and eighteen seconds to be precise," Mr. Spock interjected.

"Commander Spock, I need to get your shirt off so that I can inspect that wound more closely."

My patient raised one eyebrow, but didn't move.

"Surely you are aware, Dr. Barnes, that Mr. Spock never takes his shirt off or exposes his arms, except at the time of Ponn Far and that is not due for five more years. I, however, will be delighted to remove my shirt, particularly if your lovely nurse comes back. I'll take her over Yeoman Rand any day."

"I don't believe that my inspecting *your* body will do anything for your friend's injury. Tell me again what happened, Mr. Spock?"

"We, that is, the Enterprise, were attacked by a band of interplanetary fighters. We were in pursuit of a Romulan vessel we suspected of attacking one of our outposts along the neutral zone. Unfortunately, we encountered an energy surge which then drew us into a wormhole, which then deposited us in a completely unknown area of space. We were accosted by a trio of interplanetary fighters when we emerged. We did our best to defend ourselves, but they managed to escape. We pursued him through some sort of portal which deposited the lot of us here on Earth."

After finishing his story, Mr. Spock pulled up his shirt just enough for me to get a proper look at his wound. It was about twenty centimeters long, but clean, with dark, dried, green blood along its edges.

These conventioneers go all out, I thought, *green blood and everything.* I pulled out my stethoscope and listened to his lungs, which were clear, and his heart, but the heart sounds were barely audible.

"If you are trying to auscultate my heart, you would do better to listen here," he informed while pointing to an area in the right upper abdomen.

"Oh, yes," I replied, nonchalantly, "I guess I forgot my Vulcan anatomy. I think I missed that lecture in medical school."

I listened to the area he had pointed to and heard his heart, clear and loud, chugging along at a rate of one hundred thirty.

"Seems a little tachycardic," I observed.

"It's actually a bit slow for a Vulcan."

"And just how did you get this injury, Commander Spock? A phaser blast?"

"I believe the weapon is called a light saber. We pursued the fighters to a venue not far from here. I confronted their leader, a tall being, more machine than creature according to my tricorder..."

His voice suddenly trailed off; I turned to see Captain Kirk gesturing, signaling for Mr. Spock to remain quiet.

"Light Saber certainly fits with the injury. I'll clean it up as best I can, but you probably should see a surgeon soon."

"That should be in one hour thirty nine minutes and four seconds, although, Dr. Barnes, your skills seem far superior to our ship's surgeon."

"Thank you, but, quoting Dr. McCoy, I'm just an old country doctor."

Mr. Spock raised his other eyebrow, but did not respond. After dressing his wound I turned and saw Captain Kirk with his shirt off. He had a coy look on his face.

"Dr. Barnes," he inquired, "do you think you could convince that nurse to come give me a shot? Maybe, right in the cheek, if you get my drift?"

I gave him a long stare and handed him his shirt.

"She prefers the quiet intellectual type, Captain, sorry."

"It's in my contract, you know," he informed me with a slight leer on his face. "Paragraph twelve, section three states that I will remove my shirt at least every other episode and that sixty percent of the time I get the girl."

"This isn't Star Fleet and Miss James is never anything but professional and *never* fraternizes with her patients, Captain. So, you may put your shirt on while I attend to Mr. Spock."

I checked my tray of instruments, poured some antiseptic in one of the cups and filled the other with Lidocaine.

"I'm not sure if I'll be able to close this up, Commander," I stated as I began to cleanse the wound.

"I am sure that your efforts will be far superior to the norm, Dr. Barnes," Spock replied.

"I don't know, I'm in Internal Medicine, not surgery."

I started to inject some local but my hand was stopped by the strong grip of my patient.

"Not necessary, Dr. Barnes."

I could see him gritting his teeth, however. But, I carried on, lightly trimming away dead tissue and then doing my best to close the gaping wound.

"Where is Captain Surgery when you need him," I muttered to myself.

"Did you say something, Dr. Barnes?" Spock asked.

"Oh… no, there we go, all done."

I pushed my stool away and stood up, admiring my handiwork. The stitches were even and symmetric, the wound closed in a neat straight line.

At that moment the door to the exam room burst open and my other patient, Lord Vader, entered, accompanied by his Storm Trooper sidekicks. I was sure I heard his Star Wars theme song as he raised his light saber. Spock and Kirk jumped back, simultaneously drawing their phasers. The storm troopers crouched at Vader's side, blasters ready. I stood in the middle of this gunfight.

"Now can't you…" but before I could finish a beam shot out from Captain Kirk's phaser, not more than two inches from my nose. Darth Vader smoothly fired up his light saber and deflected the beam into the wall where it left a gaping hole with smoking blackened edges. Prudency won out over foolish bravery as I dove under the exam table, just managing to dodge a shot from a Storm

Trooper blaster.

At this moment Miss James opened the door and stuck her head in to check out the ruckus. Phaser beams and energy blasts shot back and forth while Vader skillfully deflected beams from side to side. Pockmarks of smoke and flame dotted the walls as the battle progressed, but neither side suffered any casualties. It was just after Miss James entered, before she knew what was happening, that I heard a scream and glanced up to see Miss James pouring blood out from a gaping wound where her right arm used to be. The arm, meanwhile, lay on the floor, fingers still twitching.

Despite phasers and light sabers and blasters, I jumped up and yelled as loud as I could, "LOOK AT WHAT YOU'VE DONE, YOU MONSTERS, AFTER ALL WE DID FOR YOU. STOP THIS INSTANT."

They all looked startled as I jumped to Miss James and bent down and scooped up her arm.

"You should all be ashamed of yourselves. What are you fighting about, anyway? Good versus evil? To tell you the truth I don't see a difference."

Vader looked at me as his light saber retracted. "The Force is strong in you, Dr. Barnes. You don't realize the power you could wield if you would give yourself over to It."

"To be like you? A shell of a man existing inside a black suit of armor, pretending to be big and powerful? I don't think so." I looked at Kirk and Spock. "And you two, can you make this right? Undo the damage you've done? You zoom from here to there, playing God, yet never taking any of the responsibility that a God must assume. Star Fleet, my ass. Your wonderful Star Fleet is no better than Vader's Empire. You speak about 'the Prime Directive' yet break it on every episode. Why don't you all just leave, go back to your own place and time."

At that moment I heard a familiar whine, the sound of people materializing from a transporter. I recognized Dr. McCoy and Mr. Scott, along with some red-shirted security officers (who I'm sure were destined to die sooner or later).

"Better late than never, Mr. Scott," Kirk remarked.

I turned away from the Enterprise crew, only to see that Darth Vader and his Storm Troopers were gone. I looked plaintively at Dr. McCoy.

"Doctor McCoy, Bones, do you think you can help Miss James?" I pleaded. I was cradling her head in my lap as she lapsed into unconsciousness, on the verge of shock.

McCoy looked at the severed arm and the wound at the end of her arm, which was no longer bleeding. "I'm just an old country doctor and I can't perform miracles," he said, "but, we need to get her to the ship if there is to be any chance.

"Right," I answered. "just let me close the Clinic and we can be off."

I saw Kirk looking at Spock and McCoy, shaking his head. Anger and frustration welled up inside me.

"I know what you're thinking," I stated, trying to remain calm. "Don't get involved, don't do anything to upset the status quo of what has happened or is supposed to happen. Well, your coming here may have already done that. Meanwhile, Miss James is in dire straits, she may be dying. Are you going to let that happen? Could you live with yourselves? Therefore, unless you can show me some compelling evidence which can convince me that nothing should be done and we should let Miss James suffer, you *must* do something to help."

At that moment Kirk's communicator chimed. "Let the fighters go, Mr. Sulu. We have another problem. Transporter room, we have six to beam up and have a medical team standing by."

I felt a bit of trepidation at the thought of my molecules being disassembled and then reassembled. After all it was just a television show, one that was cancelled after three seasons. But, the familiar whine started and I was soon standing in the Enterprise transporter, still supporting Miss James. Her severed arm was in a plastic garbage bag, which was inside a second bag filled with ice.

The medical crew loaded her and her arm onto a waiting stretcher and she was whisked off to sick bay, myself and Dr. McCoy at her side.

"It will be an honor and a true learning experience to watch you in action, Doctor," I said to "Bones."

He had a grave, almost worried look on his face and his hand was shaking.

"You have done this before, Doctor? I mean I did see you restore Spock's brain and patch up a badly injured Horta. Surely, reimplanting an arm is a common procedure in the twenty third century."

He just looked at me blankly.

Miss James was placed on the table and her arm placed on a second table.

"Prepare the patient, Nurse Chapel," Dr. McCoy ordered. The look of worry returned and his hand was shaking even more. I became more concerned. I'd seen the same expression on the faces of newly minted doctors on their first day of internship, but never on a veteran, seasoned surgeon. I took McCoy aside.

"Are you OK, Doctor McCoy?" I inquired, doing my best to keep the alarm out of my voice.

"It's just that there are so many structures, arteries, nerves, muscle and it's been so long. I'm just an old country doctor. That's all I ever really was supposed to be, not a super ship's surgeon. We're not meant to flit about the galaxy. It's not right; I'm just an old country..."

I cut him off, realizing he would never be able to perform such an operation, or any operation, for that matter. I was about to tell the Captain to return us to Earth when I heard a voice.

"Use the Force, Dr. Barnes. You are a doctor; you can do the surgery. The Force will be with you."

"Obiwan Kenobi?"

"The Force is strong in you, Dr. Barnes. Prepare for the surgery and let the Force guide your hand."

More and more bizarre.

OK, here goes nothing. I stepped up to the OR table and looked at the stump of Miss James severed arm and the detached arm. I put on the operating visor which should have been on Dr. McCoy and, suddenly, the operative field became clear. The computer within the visor neatly illuminated each structure: brachial artery, humerus, basilic vein, biceps muscle, and every other structure became neatly color coded and labeled.

At least the anatomy won't be difficult, but how am I to put each little vessel and fiber back together.

"Let your mind go, free yourself and rely on the Force," Obiwan suggested.

Well, I was no surgeon, that's for sure. I'd only had a twelve-week clerkship and I'd spent most of that time trying to pick up nurses in the ER.

I turned off the operating visor and put on a blinder. I thought about better times with Miss James and tried to think about nothing at all; trying to remember what Luke Skywalker had done when he blew up the first Death Star.

"Give yourself over to the Dark Side, young doctor. You don't know the power you can wield."

"GET OUT, GET OUT," I shouted in my head, trying to remove Vader from my thoughts.

Miss James, Miss James filled my head, the image of her loveliness and all the time we'd worked together.

I sensed my hands dancing across the table, working rapidly, sewing sealing, cleaning, injecting. Vessel sealant here, neural stimulation there, osteoblastic compound, more sealant, dermal regenerator, all sorts of twenty-third century medical instruments and therapies I had never thought could ever exist were employed as the Force and I worked wonders. I was oblivious to everything else until I announced: "Finished."

Miss James sat up and clenched her hand into a fist.

"Remarkable!" "Wonderful!" "Amazing!" were some of the accolades that were shouted from the many observers. I gave Miss James a hug and then sat down, finally realizing I was exhausted from the ordeal.

"I think it's time to send the two of you back," Captain Kirk announced. "But, before you go, there is one more thing to be done. Mr. Spock..."

How could I go back? Knowing what I knew. How could I ever go back to the knives and sutures of twenty-first century medicine?

It was then that Mr. Spock approached me and Miss James.

"I shall be forever grateful to you, Dr. Barnes, for repairing my injury in such a skillful manner and for teaching me, teaching all of us, about what is truly important."

And he put his hands on myself and Miss James and I heard him mutter, "Forget, forget."

We found ourselves back in the clinic. It was 6:45, just about quitting time. Miss James acted like nothing had happened. I however, did remember. I looked at her arm. It looked perfectly normal. I checked out the exam room, every charred, burned out hole in the wall had been repaired. It was as if nothing had happened. And maybe it hadn't. No one would ever believe such a story.

I turned to Miss James.

"Breakfast?" I asked.

Night Clinic Artist

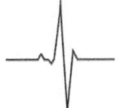

"I'M HERE AGAIN, READY FOR ANOTHER ADVENTURE INTO Never Never Land," I announced as I blasted through the door which led to the Clinic work station.

"You have some nerve showing up here," Miss James remarked. "I waited for two hours outside the concert hall. It's too bad, you missed a great show." There was a touch of venom in her voice.

"Didn't you get my message? I'm sure I sent one. Dr. Mercal sent over a sick lady from his office. It was too much for the intern to handle, so I was stuck."

"No, I didn't get any message. And then I expected you to at least show up at my apartment afterwards."

"I didn't finish with that patient until two a.m. She turned out to have *Legionella* and a perforated ulcer. Couldn't find the surgery attending for two hours. It was Bastrock, of course, probably off with one of his floozies. I wouldn't mind so much if he was a better surgeon, but his patients always have problems. I wish they would take him off the call roster. I'm sorry, love. I'll make it up to you, I promise."

"And, one more thing. Have you made a decision yet? My lease is up in six weeks, you know. They're pestering me to renew."

"You know I wouldn't stay in that apartment any longer, no matter what. It's too small and drafty and all the appliances are pretty much on their last legs."

"True, true, but the price sure is right. Anyway, it's time to get to work. Caleb the artist is in Two; severe headache."

"Caleb the artist? Should I know him?"

"Probably not personally, although you probably know his work. He's a street artist around here; he's done murals and such on the sides of most of the buildings. I think he's quite talented. He did this sketch for me while he was waiting."

Miss James held up a drawing in pencil of our clinic, the light over the door, the neon word "Open" in the window along with the sign hanging over the door which read "Clinic." Our storefront clinic stood out from the buildings around the neighborhood. Even in that sketch there was something that shouted, "Come here and be made whole." I looked forward to meeting this Caleb.

I knocked on the door and went into Exam Room Two and announced my presence in the usual way.

"Good evening, Mr...." I glanced at his chart. The only name was Caleb, no address, no phone number, just a single name.

I stumbled a bit, "Uh, Caleb, I'm Dr. Barnes. What brought you in here today?"

He didn't reply immediately. The room was darker than usual. The only light was from the X-ray box, which provided a soft illumination. Caleb was facing the far wall, his arm dancing back and forth. I noticed a long ponytail, leather jacket, and blue jeans. He ignored me and kept on working, creating a mural on our blank exam room wall. After about a minute he turned around.

"Hello, Dr. Barnes. I'm Caleb. I hope you can help me."

"I will certainly do my best," I responded, doing my best to put some concern in my voice, while trying to get a glimpse at the newly created artwork, which now adorned our previously sparse exam room. Caleb wore dark glasses and a white bandana around his head. He put out his hand, which I took, receiving a strong handshake. I glanced down at his fingers, which were long and smooth.

"What is the problem you are having?" I asked.

"I've had this headache for about two weeks. I assumed it was nothing, but it hasn't gone away."

"Where do you feel it most?"

"Right in front, like someone is boring into my brain. The light makes it worse."

"Have you tried taking anything? Tylenol, Motrin?"

"I've taken some expired Ibuprofen which helps a little bit, maybe for about an hour, but then it comes back. It seems better in the mornings when I first get up, but by afternoon I can barely move it's so bad sometimes."

"Any other medical problems? Heart, kidney, abdominal pain, nausea, vomiting, fever, weight loss?"

"No."

"Take any medications, any allergies, rash, blurred vision, or any visual changes?"

"No, except the light bothers me."

"OK, OK. Let me check you. I need to turn on the light."

"Go ahead, I'll be OK."

"Let me check a few things with the lights off first."

I took out my flashlight and shined it in his eyes. His pupils reacted briskly.

"I'm no Opthamologist and I haven't done this since fourth year, but I'll give it a try. I picked up the opthalmoscope and aimed it towards his eyes. I was greeted by the red reflex and was able to get a clear look at his retina.

Still have the old touch. But, what am I looking for?

I could see blood vessels and the optic nerve, but had no idea if any of it was pathologic.

Where's the CT Scanner when you need it?

"I'm going to turn the lights on now."

"OK," he answered, but there was a sense of apprehension, almost doom as I flicked the switch.

Caleb winced and squinted when the light came on, then put his hands to his temples and rubbed them vigorously as if he was trying to vanquish the demons that were pounding on his head.

"I'll try to be quick," I assured him as I auscultated, palpated, and inspected from head to toe. Everything was normal. I turned the light off as Miss James stuck her head in the room.

"I need you in Three. An elderly man just came in, wheezing, blue lips, doesn't look too good. I put him on a hundred percent oxygen."

"Did you call for an ambulance?"

"Started to, but the man said he wouldn't go to the hospital."

"I'll be back in few minutes, Caleb. Just lay here with the lights off, that'll probably help."

I glanced at the chart outside Exam Room Three.

"Heinrich Dietrich, ninety three," I murmured as I quickly knocked and opened the door.

"Good evening, Mr. Dietrich, I'm Dr. Barnes," I started with my usual bedside banter.

I was greeted by the raspy sound of labored breathing. Mr. Dietrich was sitting upright, his chest heaving as each breath came with herculean effort. His lips were blue, his eyes sunken deep into their sockets. His skin was a grayish yellow with superficial scratches and healing sores. I understood immediately why he didn't want to go to the hospital.

"Terminal?" I asked.

He nodded in the affirmative.

"What can I do for you?"

He handed me a piece of paper and gestured for me to read it.

Chaim Fiesel, 3233 Elm, #11

"Send for him… *Please*," he requested, his voice, with a bit of an accent, a barely audible rasp.

"But, I can't…"

"*PLEASE*," this time almost a command.

I looked at the paper and then at my dying patient.

"OK," I answered.

I left the room and found Miss James at the nurse's station.

"Anything else waiting?" I asked, sort of nonchalantly.

"Quiet as a mouse. What's going on in Three?"

"Mr. Deitrich has terminal cancer. He's dying and he knows it. He asked me to find this man, a Chaim Fiesel. He's supposed to be in an apartment over on Elm, only about five minutes away. I thought, maybe, one of us could run over and fetch him. You know, grant the dying man his last request."

"I'll go," she replied. "That way if anything bad comes in you can take care of it."

"I hate to let you go by yourself. It may not be safe."

"I'll be OK. I know that apartment building. It has a big, mean, Rottweiler watchdog and is pretty secure. It should only take a few minutes, assuming Mr. Fiesel is there and will come with me."

She was out the door in thirty seconds and I manned the front desk. A woman came in with her child suffering from an earache. They were quickly examined, diagnosed, treated and out the door. I went back to check on Caleb. He was up on a chair, creating a new masterpiece on the wall. All I could make out in the dim light were shades of black, gray, and white.

I heard the door open and saw Miss James and a short, bent, elderly man come in. He was dressed in a dark gray suit, wore thick glasses, and had a dark gray moustache. His eyes however, were alive, a vibrant blue. I hurried to meet them.

"Dr. Barnes, this is Mr. Fiesel," she reported as the man put out his hand. I noticed the fingers were bent and twisted.

"Nice to meet you," I said, taking his hand in mine, giving him a strong greeting. "Did the lovely Miss James explain the situation?"

"She did, she did," he answered, his voice marked by an Eastern European accent, not much different from Mr. Dietrich's. "I do not know this Heinrich Dietrich and I do not know why he would ask for me. Perhaps, you can find out more?"

"I'll go ask," I replied. "Maybe he's a long lost relative and wants to leave you some money. He is dying, you know."

"Yes, yes, Miss James did tell me that."

I returned to Room Three. Mr. Dietrich seemed a bit more comfortable.

"Mr. Fiesel is here, but he is wondering why you asked for him. He says he does not know you."

"It's true, he does not, but in a way he does. Tell him I must see him. I must tell him I'm sorry."

"Sorry? Sorry for what," I had to ask. "I ask you because I know that he will ask me."

"Sorry for what I did, to him, to his people, during the war at Dachau."

Now it was clear to me. Mr. Dietrich, with his clearly German accent. Mr. Fiesel, a Jew, also German, perhaps a survivor of one of the camps, all adding up to a search for peace on one's deathbed.

"I'll carry your message to him," I whispered in Mr. Dietrich's ear.

I hope Fiesel understands.

I went back to the lobby where Mr. Fiesel was waiting and explained the situation. Fiesel's face turned red as he heard my report.

"I was in Dachau; my whole family, mother, father, two sisters, died at Dachau. He may have been their executioner, for all I know," his voice was growing louder. "I should hear the confession of a murderer, a man who served in a place that took my whole life from me? No, I will not. I cannot."

"But surely you can find it within yourself to forgive, to give this man some peace before he goes?" Miss James asked.

But Fiesel said nothing. He sat down and stared at his gnarled hands.

"I was a violinist," he said softly. "I started playing at the age of two. I was the youngest performer ever with the Munich Symphony. But, they took that from me." His voice started to rise and tremble. "Look at these hands, look at what they did to my hands. First they smashed my violin into a million splinters, then they smashed my hands."

And I saw his broken hands, reflections of a broken soul. I left him and returned to the dying Dietrich, but first I saw a light coming from Exam Roon One. I had almost forgotten about Caleb. I opened the door and saw him sitting up in the chair. And, I saw his finished mural. It was a scene of horror. A death camp surrounded by barbed wire, emaciated bodies withering away and dying while soldiers brandishing rifles watched, laughed, and did nothing. The sky was filled with black clouds, which matched the blackness of death in that camp. Except at the end of the mural there was a bit of yellow, a sliver of sunlight which illuminated a corner of the camp where one soldier was stooping down, giving a red apple to a boy. The boy was like the rest of the prison, wasted, dying, dressed in a ragged striped uniform.

I felt a body brush up against me. I turned, expecting to see Miss James, and was a bit surprised to see Mr. Fiesel, tears were streaming down his face. He looked up at me and then left me and went into Exam Room Three.

I continued to stare at that mural adorning the room's previously empty wall. It was a masterpiece of death and hope. The blacks and grays, the ominous clouds, the pall of death which hung over that camp were all overshadowed by the small expression of kindness set off to one side. In the midst of all that despair, one glimmer of hope shined through. I turned to offer my critique to Caleb, but he was gone.

Mr. Fiesel emerged from Room Three shaking his head, but also smiling.

"You see," I began to comment, "a bit of forgiveness..."

He held up his hand to stop me. Miss James stood at my side to hear his story.

"You don't understand, Dr. Barnes, neither of you do. This picture, this vision of death with its small ray of light illuminating a solitary act of human decency is not just an abstract artist's interpretation. All that death, all those guards and barbed wire is exactly as it was. And, that soldier giving the apple to that little boy is real. That little boy is me. Look at the date on the picture: September 13, 1943. I remember that day; it was my birthday. I turned ten on that day. I was so hungry, I thought I wouldn't live for another minute if I didn't get something to eat. One of the guards took pity on me. He was about to eat an apple and must have seen me staring at him. He smiled at me and then got up and *came to me*. He bent over and gave me that apple and, along with it, gave me the hope and will to survive. You see, I was all alone; my family was gone, murdered by the Nazis. All I could hope for was death, disease, and despair. But, he gave me hope and I did survive. I never became the musician I should have been, the Nazi's made sure of that, but I did come to this country and became an art dealer. This picture reminded me that in the midst of hatred and chaos and evil, human kindness might still exist."

"Is that why you changed your mind? To pass on this human kindness?" I asked.

"Maybe," he answered, "but there is even more. Look at the image closely, look at the helmet."

We bent over and stared at the soldier and saw clearly on the brim of the helmet the letters HD.

"Heinrich Dietrich, the dead man in your exam room is the soldier in this mural. He gave me his apple and a second chance at life and I had to thank him. You know, Dr. Barnes, he lived only two blocks from me for over thirty years but I never realized it and he could never gather the courage to come to me. He told me now he would walk past my art gallery; he did this hundreds of times. He even found the courage to come inside once. He asked for me, but when I came out he had left. When I saw him today I knew him immediately. He asked my forgiveness. He offered no explanations or rationalizations. He knew what was done, what he had done, how he had helped it all happen and how he had done nothing to stop it. Yet through all that evil, there still existed this one tiny shred of humanity."

We three stared at the painting for a bit longer.

"Where is the artist?" Fiesel asked. "I would like to meet him and thank him personally."

"Caleb; he must have left. He lives somewhere in this neighborhood, I'm not sure exactly where. I'm sure you've seen his work all around. He has created murals, like this one, all over the city."

"I have seen them, it is truly remarkable work, a wonderful talent, but, perhaps in need of a little guidance," Fiesel murmured. "I will have to search for him. After all, I am an art dealer."

He shook my hand and gave Miss James a light peck on her cheek and went away.

It was coming up on seven when he left, almost the end of our shift.

"What should we do with this mural?" I wondered. "I don't think it is quite right for a medical clinic."

"Death, despair, and hope?" Miss James said out loud. "Isn't that what we deal in here?"

"Perhaps... but not in that order," I observed.

"I'll tell you what," she replied. "I'll call up Fiesel later today and ask him if he wants it for his gallery. I'm sure he can figure out a way to get it from here to there."

I snapped a photo of the mural, just in case it was somehow lost, and then we went back to the nursing station and found a final gift from Caleb.

On the desk was another picture, bright and colorful. It was my apartment. Seated on the couch were two people, myself and Miss James. There was an open door, which showed the bedroom and the bathroom, with two towels on the rack and two toothbrushes hanging by the sink. Next to the drawing was a note.

My headache is gone. Thank you so much, Dr. Barnes.
—Caleb

Miss James and I stared at each other and then, almost simultaneously asked.

"How does he know?"

We didn't have an answer.

Winter Night Clinic

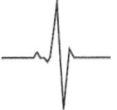

"I'VE BRAVED THE RAIN AND SLEET AND SNOW AND HAVE returned for another exciting shift here at the fabled 'Night Clinic,' " I announced as I shook the snow and slush from my boots. "Maybe the bad weather will keep it quiet."

"Don't hold your breath; all the exam rooms are full and five more waiting," Miss James reported. "You can start with the swollen ankle in One."

Her voice was cold with more than a touch of annoyance.

What did I do now? I put my dirty clothes in the laundry, washed the dishes, put the toilet seat down, let her...

"Miss James," I began, "have I done something to upset you?" I did my best to feign contriteness.

"The time is 7:30. Our shift starts at seven. Why are you always late?"

"Well, today I had to..."

She just walked away, not really interested in an answer to what I now surmised was a purely rhetorical question. Her point made, we went to work.

"Gregory Jackson, ankle injury playing basketball, nineteen, lives on Maple, unemployed," the chart reported.

I knocked twice and then went in and saw a very tall, thin young man with his ankle elevated and swathed in an ice pack.

"Good evening, Mr. Jackson, what happened to you?"

"Well, Doc, I was driving to the hoop and was about to do my Dr. J, you know fly under, up and over the hoop to slam it home when this little guy, Bennie, I think is his name, undercuts me. I landed right on my ankle and then it swelled it almost the size of the ball. The other guys almost had to carry me here."

I pulled off the ice pack and then looked at the X-rays, which were already pulled up on the screen. I blew them up as big as I could.

Soft tissue swelling, separation of the joint, nothing broken.

I looked more closely at the ankle, which was very swollen and had a slight purple hue. When I tried to move it my patient winced in pain.

"It looks like you have a very bad sprain, Mr. Jackson. I'll wrap it up for you, but you need to keep it iced down for at least the next twenty four hours and stay off if for about two weeks. I'll give you the number to the Ortho clinic at the University Hospital, call or go there to make an appointment to be seen next week, OK?"

"Got it, Doc. Oh, by the way, can you get me the number or address for Medusa?"

"Excuse me?"

"I saw her go into one of your exam rooms, this chick we call Medusa. We see her around all the time, but she won't talk to anyone. But, she's one hot chick. Every guy I know wants to get 'in' with her, if you get my drift."

"Sorry, you're out of luck. You'll just have to do that on your own. Just check out with Miss James at the desk. She'll have all the instructions and the number to call for follow up written down for you."

I went on to Room Two, but I did glance at the chart for Room Three. Sure enough the name was Medusa, while the rest of the chart was blank. First, however, there was abdominal pain in Two.

I glanced at the name, Rufus T. Horsefly, fifty five, abdominal pain for two days.

"Good evening, Mr. Horsefly. I'm Dr. Barnes," I began, trying not to betray my desire to dispatch him and his abdominal pain as quickly as possible so that I could move on to this mysterious Medusa. "What is the problem you're having?"

"Hello, Dr. Barnes," he answered as I sat down across from him. "I've had this pain in my stomach and back for two days."

"How did it start?" I asked, trying not to look too bored.

"It started in my back then moved to the front. Today I had some numbness in my legs and I almost passed out. I figured I better get it checked out, you know, better safe than sorry."

I was actually beginning to get worried at this point and, as it turned out, with good reason. I quickly gathered the rest of his history: untreated hypertension, cigarette smoking, some alcohol use, father died suddenly at age sixty.

"Let me check you now," I requested/commanded. He lay down on the exam table and I felt his abdomen. He cringed slightly as I palpated all over his abdomen, particularly just above his umbilicus as I felt what I feared, the prominent thump, thump, thump of what I presumed was an abdominal aortic aneurysm. I felt his femoral pulses, which were only barely palpable, while his carotid and radial pulses were strong. I looked at the chart again, recorded blood pressure was 180/95, heart rate was sixty.

"Miss James, call 911 please and request an ambulance," I called out to her at the front desk. I started an IV on Mr. Horsefly and drew some tubes of blood to go with him for a type and cross and lab.

"Mr. Horsefly," I started to explain, "you almost certainly have an abdominal aortic aneurysm, either expanding or already ruptured. This is a very serious condition, one which is life threatening. An ambulance is on the way to take you to the hospital where you will need some sort of surgery. Do you understand?"

The look on his face told me everything as his lighthearted countenance was replaced by fear.

"I'm going to call the hospital and ask that Dr. Singer be standing by; he's the best vascular surgeon around, OK?"

He nodded his head and I left the room. Luckily, Dr. Singer was available and I was able to speak to him directly. The ambulance arrived and Mr. Horsefly was wheeled out to the waiting vehicle, lights flashing in the snow, siren ready to sing.

As he was leaving, I had to lighten the moment a bit, "Mr. Horsefly, by the way. In the movie Duck Soup, Groucho's name is Rufus T. Firefly, not Horsefly."

Mr. Horsefly smiled as they were loading him into the ambulance.

"I know, 'The horseflies were on the Firefly's and the Firefly's were on the Mayflower,' " were his parting words as they loaded him in the back. I made a mental note to check on him the next day.

Back to the grind, and Medusa.

I knocked on the door and entered Room Three.

"Good evening, Miss..." I started my usual introduction but stopped when I saw the young woman waiting inside.

She was sitting on the chair, dressed in a very thin coat, her legs were bare and she had her arms wrapped around her chest. She wore ragged boots with a hole in the bottom. She had long black hair with a white bandana and her skin was the color of chocolate mousse, smooth and silky. Her eyes, those eyes were the most amazing eyes I'd ever seen, dark brown with long lashes. All in all, even as dirty and disheveled as she was, she was an amazing, striking beauty. I caught myself and started my introduction again.

"Miss Medusa, I am Dr. Barnes. What is the problem that brings you in here tonight?"

"Cold," was all she said.

I was caught a bit off guard by the brevity of her answer. "Excuse me, did you say that you have a cold?" I asked.

"No, I was cold and needed a place to warm up," her voice was as silky smooth as her skin and there was an aura about her which beckoned to draw me into her world. I had to stop myself and even shake my head to return my focus to medicine.

"I'm sorry, but this Clinic is for those who are sick or injured. I know it's unusually cold tonight and wet and dreary, but there are other places you can go. There are shelters and there is the mission over on Fourteenth Street."

"I can't go to those places. Bad things happen to me. Oh, why did I ever come to this place and *time?* I never should have been so trusting."

Her words started to pique my interest. "Place and time?" She certainly was not the Medusa known from mythology. No snakes for hair or gnarly face and teeth. Indeed, she was the complete opposite. There was great beauty, which radiated from her and filled the room, and that aura, a remarkable feeling which emanated from her soul, reached out and touched me. She did seem to be in some sort of trouble, but a chief complaint of "cold" did not require my medical services. However, the profound sense of sadness which surrounded her, as well as the inexplicable attraction I was beginning to feel, overwhelmed any necessity to follow the book.

"We are sort of busy, but you can stay in our break room for a little while. You can warm up and I'll see if we can find a better place for you to go."

Maybe my apartment. No, no, don't forget Miss James.

"Thank you," she replied.

I led her to the back of the Clinic, got her a cup of coffee and a blanket.

"Tea, please, if it's not too much trouble," she requested, but to me it seemed to be more than a simple request. I fixed her a cup of tea, English Breakfast, from the supply that Miss James kept and started to go back to work, but I almost couldn't drag myself away from her. Finally, the slightly irritated voice of Miss James snapped me back to reality.

"Dr. Barnes, patients are ready in Rooms One, Two, Three, and Four, and the waiting room is full."

I felt a jolt back to reality.

"I must go," I said to Medusa, "but I *will* come back and check on you when I can."

"Thank you, Doctor," she replied, clutching the mug of tea tightly in two hands,

I picked up the chart for Room One, Mo Smith, lacerated arm. I knocked on the door and went in to find Mr. Smith sprawled out on the table, a towel soaked in blood covering his left arm.

"Good Evening Mr. Smith, what happened…"

And so it went, Room One, then Two, then Three, Four, back to One and on and on; diarrhea, fever, back pain, headache, belly pain, broken ankle, broken arm, broken hand, until it was four a.m.

"Just one more patient, Dr. Barnes, waiting in Room Two," Miss James reported. "A Mr. Persy, sore neck."

"Thank you, Nurse. I think I've earned my money tonight. How many patients have I seen?"

"Forty eight. Mr. Persy will make forty nine. I think that's a record. The cold weather brings them in, I think," She concluded.

I knocked on Room Two and went inside.

"Good morning, Mr. Persy. I'm Dr. Barnes. What is the problem you are having?"

"Is she here?"

"Is who here?"

"Medusa. I've been searching for her for quite a while."

What does HIPAA say?

"I'm sorry, Mr. Persy, but I do not know any 'Medusa' and if I did and she was a patient, I would not be allowed to tell you; rules you know."

I wasn't sure why I didn't give him some intimation that I had at least seen her. Technically, she had not been a patient, just cold and all I had treated her with was a cup of tea.

Maybe I can learn more.

"Perhaps, if you could tell me something about her, I could help you. She may have passed through here under an assumed name. It has been known to happen before. After all, we are here to help people who are ill or injured. All we want to do is make them better. Most of the time we don't care if the name is real."

He scratched his head and then stroked his chin.

"OK, let me tell you about her. Medusa was born in what would be modern day Turkey, a long time ago. Nothing is known about her parents, but she had two sisters, both of whom are dead. They were all hideously ugly and the two sisters pined away, wishing to be beautiful, like Medusa. Medusa, however, was a real beauty, but this beauty was more of a curse.

"She is most beautiful," I blurted out, before I realized I'd blown her cover.

Mr. Persy smiled before he continued. "As I stated, she was a beauty. But, Medusa, ah, sweet Medusa, she was always lost in her thoughts. She could read and write and could remember every little detail of everything she had ever seen, heard, or done. And, more than anything, she was wise. From the time she was twelve years old, barely an adult, people came to her for advice.

"Kings would come and ask if they should go to war or surrender. Men would ask about marrying, women would ask if they should accept proposals. When was the best time to plant, if the rains would be coming, and on and on. And, she was not clairvoyant, just wise. She had a way of sifting through a mountain of information and distilling it down to its essentials and then rendering precise and accurate judgment. This was a gift from the gods. Being human she could not help but boast. She was reported to have said she was wiser than Zeus and Athena."

"Wait," I interjected, "are you telling me that she has been around for thousands of years. That the Medusa who is or was sitting in my little break room, drinking tea and wrapped in one of my blankets, is the same Medusa from Greek mythology?"

"Yes," was his terse reply, "but she is far different from the beast depicted in the mythology."

"That is for sure," I answered, "but, I should not have interrupted. Please go on with your story."

"Medusa is and always has been the epitome of beauty, grace, charm, the perfect embodiment of womanhood. You have, I'm sure, seen her, been with her and felt the strange allure. That is Medusa. Think of history, the great beauties men have given their very being to possess; women that men have fought and died for: Helen of

Troy, Nefirtiti, Bathsheba, and how many other nameless women. She was all of them. Medusa was Solomon's favorite concubine, coming to his chamber night after night; she was consort to Roman Emperors, Arthur's Guinevere, and so many more. She is ageless and she is timeless, yet through it all she suffers."

"Suffers?" I asked. "I would have thought she would have everything she could want, but, from what I've seen, she has nothing."

"Of course she has nothing. She wants nothing but to be alone, to be removed from the curse?"

"I still don't understand," I had to admit.

"That is because all you see is a beautiful woman and in your mind beauty opens many doors. You feel the intoxication, but don't see that there is a person there. I, on the other hand, know what she wants all too well and I can help free her from her sorrow. I have pursued her for all these years, because I want to take her away and free her from her burden."

I listened closely, not sure if any of it was true or if this Mr. Persy was merely a pimp trying to get his hooker to tow the line.

After a bit of thought and reflection, I knew that it was up to Medusa to make some sort of decision.

"Wait here, Mr. Persy," I instructed.

I went back to our break room. Medusa was still there, still wrapped in the blanket, sitting on the chair with her arms holding her knees tightly to her chest, slowly rocking back and forth.

"I'm still cold," she cooed and then she gave me her smile and I knew why men throughout the ages would fight and die over her. But, my professional demeanor took over.

"There's a man here looking for you, Medusa. He says his name is Mr. Persy. Do you know him?" I asked softly.

I put my hand on her shoulder and she pulled away and shook her head violently back and forth.

"NO, NO, and NO," she shouted. "DON'T LET HIM, DON'T LET HIM, PLEASE!"

I saw the fear of the caged animal in her eyes as the door burst open and Mr. Persy entered.

"Medusa, my Medusa, you've eluded me for so long, but now I've found you, alone, and I will have my victory. I will fulfill the task set before me and she will be mine forever," Persy hissed.

"You're mad, Perseus. She's been dead for thousands of years. No matter what you do to me you can't have her. She's probably nothing but dust by now, dirt which has grown up to become grass, then consumed by some lowly animal, a cow perhaps, or a bull, or the Minotaur. Yes, consumed and digested and rejected like dung. That's all your precious Andromeda is; Minotaur dung and that's all you deserve."

Miss James came in to check out all the commotion, startling Mr. Persy, that is Perseus, and I took the opportunity to step between Medusa and Perseus, but the crazed Greek "hero" pushed us all away, reached into his overcoat and pulled out a very long, very sharp gleaming knife.

"There is no help for you here. No king's guards to protect you, no smitten Alexander to offer you refuge. Only these pitiful mortals. I'll have your head and my happiness. Andromeda will be free and we will fly away together."

He moved closer towards Medusa, his knife held high.

I heard a loud thump in the waiting room.

Maybe it's the police or a disgruntled patient tired of waiting.

There was a loud crash as the door to the break room ripped away from its hinges and fell to the floor. A sleek white horse bolted through, its black eyes determined, white wings sprouted from its back as it reared up and brought its front legs down on Perseus, knocking him to the floor and then kicking him to the side like the piece of garbage he truly was.

Pegasus.

The winged horse bounded towards Medusa and she effortlessly climbed on its back. The powerful beast kicked a huge hole in the back wall and the two rode off into the east towards the just rising sun. A faint glow arose from horse and Mistress as the snow fell around them and they made their escape. Miss James and I stood silently and watched.

"Perseus," I exclaimed.

He was up on his feet, brandishing his knife at us.

"I have no quarrel with either of you. But, if you should ever see her, call me. The things I told you are all true. What she said is mere fantasy; the product of a deranged mind. I bid you farewell."

He left a card on the table and stepped towards the opening in the wall.

"But, let us check you. You may be seriously injured. Pegasus' kick packs quite a wallop."

"I have lived for all these thousands of years and suffered far greater injury than a trifling kick from an old nag."

He stepped through the hole in the wall and was gone. I looked up to see him flying towards the east, his boots had wings.

Like Hermes' boots.

I turned away and looked into my companion's eyes.

"Do you believe any of this, Miss James?" I asked.

"What's not to believe? There is a big hole in the wall and then there is him."

"Him?"

She gestured for me to look behind and there, standing in the doorway, was the Minotaur. He was dressed in a black suit and had a gold ring on his finger, but there was no doubt as to the beast's identity.

"This is not some sort of Halloween gag, is it? Because, trick or treat and Halloween were months ago."

"I'm sorry," the monster apologized, speaking impeccable English with a slight accent. "I saw that you're light was on and that you were open, so I thought you might be able to help me. You see I have this rash…"

"Miss James, would please take Mr. Minotaur…"

"Just the Minotaur, if you please. It commands more respect."

"Would you please take the Minotaur to Room One? I'll be there in a few minutes."

What time is it? Isn't this shift over yet? Five thirty, an hour and a half to go. I guess I need to face the Minotaur.

I did remember reading something about the Minotaur recently, but the details eluded me at that moment.

I knocked on the door to Room One as I glanced at the chart: Quinton Arbus Taurus Aegus Minos, "Minotaur," DOB unknown, originally from Crete, previous neck trauma, recently hospitalized following severe exposure with dehydration, previously prolonged exposure to cold, starvation... chief complaint: rash on upper chest.

"Good evening, Minotaur, or rather, good morning. What's the problem that brings you in this fine morning?" I asked, trying to maintain my professional appearance.

"I've had this rash along my upper chest for almost two weeks now, right where my body transitions from fur to hairless skin. I've tried all the usual creams and nothing is working. It's driving me crazy," he reported, his manner polite and refined.

"You're in luck. I've been rotating through Dermatology this month. I'm pretty well up on all the rashes. Let me take a look. Does it itch a lot?"

"Horribly, day and night. I can't sleep. I thought I might have fleas, even went to the vet for a flea dip, but nothing helps."

"Well, let's take a look."

He took off his black overcoat and suit coat, followed by his white shirt and tie. There was an abrupt transition from the short, coarse hair of his bullish shoulders, neck and, head to the smooth white skin of his human half. At this changeover point the skin was red and thickened with vesicular lesions. There was some excoriation where the Minotaur had been scratching.

Very strange, very unusual indeed.

"I need to take a closer look at the hairline, but I think I know what the problem is," I informed the Minotaur. I found a magnifying glass in the exam room drawer and began a very close inspection of the beast's hair. Sure enough they were there, tiny whitish "nits" on the hair and I noticed some tiny bugs moving about.

"You, my dear Minotaur, have lice. I'm surprised the flea dip didn't help, but sometimes these tiny monsters can be very tenacious. Give me some time and I'll do my best to get rid of most of them. It might be best to shave a lot of your hair, particularly along this transition zone. But, first you'll need a shampoo."

Lice was a fairly common complaint at the Clinic and we maintained a supply of medicated shampoo which usually worked well to kill any adult forms of the vermin. I gave him a vigorous lathering, let it sit for a bit, and then rinsed.

Next, I pulled out a fine comb and began going through all his hair, brushing away some of the whitish eggs, while pulling out hairs that stubbornly held on to their cargo. This, I had learned over the years, was the only way to get rid of the nasty "nits" which were cemented to his hair.

"While I'm working, Minotaur, I was wondering if you know anything about Medusa and Perseus? I assume you were around during their time. What is the truth?"

"A sad story, that's for sure. The events actually took place before my birth, but I did get a firsthand account from one of the old guards in Minos' palace before I was locked away in the Labyrinth.

"Medusa always had amazing beauty, but also intelligence and wisdom. So beautiful, in fact, that all the lady "gods" were jealous. They concocted the story which has become the myth which has survived all these years. Medusa, one of three Gorgons, was supposed to be so ugly that anyone who looked at her would be turned to stone. She had hair which was snakes and eyes which turned anyone who gazed into them to stone. This kept most everyone away. But, this was not enough for Athena and Aphrodite. They were so jealous of her that they plotted to have her killed.

"Perseus was their dupe. He really did venture out on a quest to kill her and to bring her head to King Polydectes, as recounted in the myth, but, like most myths, that was the only kernel of truth in the story. The gods promised Perseus that he would have Andromeda as his bride if he could vanquish Medusa. Andromeda was young and very pretty and her father was very powerful. Perseus immediately was smitten by her charm and the prospect of ruling the land as the next king and vowed to return after he was successful.

"Perseus did manage to find Medusa with the aid of the gods. But, he first had to deal with Medusa's two sisters, who were truly ugly just as it says in the myth. Their job in life was to shield their stunning, gifted sister from unwanted visitors. Perseus was a truly great warrior, however, and he was determined to vanquish Medusa. He brutally murdered Medusa's sisters.

"He came upon the young, innocent, beautiful maiden and threatened to kill her if he did not tell him where he could find the supremely ugly Medusa. He was still expecting a Medusa with snakes for hair and hideously gnarled features, which is what the entire world assumed Medusa to be. That young maiden, who really was Medusa, realized the danger she was in and tricked Perseus. She sent him up into the hills, saying that the repulsive Medusa was in one of the caves. Perseus charged up the incline, his sword raised and his shiny shield slung over his back, ready to do battle with a monster. Meanwhile, Medusa made her escape on the back of Pegasus. And she's been on the run ever since."

"It's sad, so sad," he continued. "Medusa has only good qualities. She has to be the most beautiful and tragic woman to ever live. Meanwhile, Perseus has lived with this obsession for thousands of years. Andromeda is long dead, the Greek gods have been relegated to myth; only a few of us live on. Myself, Pandora, Perseus, Medusa, Hercules, and a few more have survived through the ages, through all the sordid years of human history.

"Pegasus, by the way, the winged horse, is Medusa's greatest friend and ally. She raised him from a colt and he is never far away from her. That is one reason she has managed to survive and escape all these years."

The Minotaur finished his story and sat while I continued to comb through his hair. Miss James, by this time, had joined me.

"Finished," I announced. "I think all the nasty little creatures and their eggs are gone. To be really thorough you could slather on some olive oil and leave it over night. That will suffocate any little beasts who may be lingering. Oh, and good luck on your new job at the University. I do remember reading about you and your remarkable life in the paper. I think you will turn the Department of Antiquities on its head."

"Thank you, Doctor and Nurse," the Minotaur answered. "I wish you well. And, don't worry about Medusa. She will be all right. Look for her, someday, on a movie screen or on the arm of a powerful senator or prince. Oh, and look for my story. I think you would enjoy it. Good morning."

And he left.

Miss James and I stared at each other, shrugged our shoulders, and waited for the next shift.

"Breakfast? Or a bath?" she asked.

"Both," I answered.

A few minutes later we left together.

Night Clinic Christmas

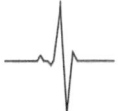

"I'M HERE, BEARING GIFTS ON THIS GLORIOUS CHRISTMAS Eve," I announced as I placed my packages on the table in the break room. "Just a few special items for my special nurse and friend."

"Only two minutes late; you're improving." Miss James remarked and then gave me her special smile.

"Christmas Eve, a new moon, fifteen degrees outside, it ought to be a quiet night," I responded. "What am I saying? I'm sure I just jinxed us."

Miss James looked at the presents, each carefully wrapped with shiny silver and gold Christmas paper.

"Oh no, you can't open them yet; not until midnight. I'll put them under the tree in the lobby."

I carried the packages to the front and placed them under the small tree, which was perched on the reception desk. There was another present there already with my name on the card.

Dear Miss James.

At that moment an elderly couple walked in, both neatly dressed, holding hands, each with a twinkle in their eyes.

"Good evening, Dr. Barnes," the man greeted me, staring at my badge. "My name is Curley and this is my wife, Cupcake. We need some help."

"Certainly, Sir, that *is* why we're here." I answered, trying to be polite. "What is the problem?"

At this moment, Miss James appeared.

"We need some basic information before we can see you, Mr..." she said before she was interrupted.

"Curley," the man replied. "Curley Fries is my full name and my wife is Red Velvet Cupcake. Give me your forms so we can get started."

He took the clipboard from Miss James and they turned to sit down in the lobby. He gave me a wink and a nod as he sat down to fill out the necessary papers, never breaking his hold of Cupcake's hand.

I went to the back while Miss James manned the reception desk. A younger man came in with a noticeable limp.

So much for a quiet night.

After a few minutes Cupcake and Curley were brought back to Exam Room One. I picked up the chart and perused their information:

Complaint: Chest Pain
Patient name: Curley Fries
Age: 87
Occupation: Song and Dance
Address: 214 Blakemore, #330
Current Medications: Lisinopril, Crestor
Allergies: none known
Do you smoke: occasional cigar
Do you drink alcohol: not to excess
Any previous surgery: none

Nothing unusual.

I gave two short knocks on the door and went inside. Curley and Cupcake were seated next to each other, still holding hands. He was thin, short, maybe five five, with white hair and thick black glasses, which magnified his sparkling eyes, and he had an infectious smile on his face. Cupcake was shorter, maybe five one, black hair with a touch of gray and very smooth skin for an elderly woman. All in all, they were a very handsome couple.

"Good evening, again, Curley and Cupcake. What is the problem that brings you in here?" I asked in my usual professional tone.

Curley jumped out of his chair and extended his hand. He grabbed mine and started shaking it effusively.

"Good evening. I'm Curley Fries and this is Cupcake, Red Velvet Cupcake to be exact. You've heard of us? No. You must be living under a rock. We've been on the circuit for over sixty years. We were very big in the Borscht Belt."

I gave him a confused look.

"The Borscht Belt, you know, the Catskills, Long Island, New Joisey. You have to say it right. Joisey. We don't tour anymore. Now it's just local weddings, Bar Mitzvahs, graduations, birthdays. Here's our card. When you and that lovely nurse finally tie the knot, don't forget about Curley and Cupcake. Oh, but I've forgotten my manners. Dr. Barnes, how nice to meet you properly. It's not often I get to meet a legend."

He offered his hand again and I shook it again.

"Legend? I think you have me confused with another Dr. Barnes. I'm just third-year medical resident trying to make a few extra dollars. Now what can I do for you?"

"You mean you're not the famous Dr. Barnes, founder of the Barnes Institute for Penile Rejuvenation? Then I'm not sure you can help us. Oh, wait, I almost forgot. I've been having pain in my chest. Right here next to my sternum. Like Zero Mostel was sitting on it."

I looked at him with a smile on my face. I was beginning to like Curley.

"How often are you getting this pain?"

"Whenever me and Cupcake have sex. Three or four times a day."

Cupcake gave her a companion a short kick.

"Tell him the truth, Curley," she demanded.

I turned to her, "What is the truth… er, Cupcake?"

"Well, the truth is we only have sex twice a day, except on Sundays, when it's three times."

They both smiled and then Curley said, "The pain comes on

when I'm active, you know, lifting, pushing. It had been happening once every couple of weeks, but yesterday and today it's been more often and lasting longer. Usually one Nitro and I'm good, but these last couple of days it's been…"

And he burst into song: "A Heartache tonight, A Heartache tonight, I know…"

"OK, OK, I get the picture. Let me check you real quick. Do you have a regular Cardiologist?"

"Dr. Steinberg, a nice Jewish doctor, really *schmart,* if you get my drift, and not a bad singer."

"Good, he's at the University. I might be able to access your records, get an old EKG."

I felt his pulse, which was strong and regular. I listened to his heart, which was loud and clear. Lungs were clear. No evidence of cardiac enlargement, pulses all strong, abdomen benign.

"You look good on exam, Curley. Miss James will be in to do an EKG and draw some blood."

"Good, good. She's a real keeper, just like Cupcake here, don't let her get away. Sixty five years tomorrow, Dr. Barnes. I've been on the lookout for a better model all these years, but nothing's come along."

And he smiled at her and took her hand in his again.

I stepped out into the hallway where I found Miss James coming out of Room Two.

"Lacerated leg. He says he cut it on some glass, but it looks like a razor to me. Pretty deep. He may need to go to the hospital," she reported.

"Thanks. EKG in One, if you can. He's been having increasing chest pain, but he looks strong as an ox. Anymore out there?"

"Too many. Shouldn't they all be going to church?"

I went into Room Two. Rodney Smith, twenty two, unemployed, no medical problems.

"Good evening, Mr. Smith. What happened to you?" I began.

"Cut myself on this metal table, Doc," he answered.

"Let me take a look," I requested as I unrolled the gauze dressing to reveal a deep laceration, almost ten inches long, on his left lateral thigh. It was straight and clean, extending to the fascia, but only about one centimeter of muscle was exposed.

"That must have been quite a metal table, Mr. Smith. I hope the other guy is OK."

"Chicken shit ran away."

"Never heard of a table running away. Never mind, we'll get this sewed up."

The tray was there, opened and ready with appropriate suture, Lidocaine and Betadine. I took off my white coat and went to work and, in what I thought was no time, had my patient sutured and bandaged and ready to go. As I left his room I heard singing from the lobby.

> "Joy to the world, the Lord is come
> Let Earth Receive her King…"

Curley and Cupcake were standing in front of what was becoming a very full waiting room, singing. I have to admit they had pretty good voices and the waiting patients looked very appreciative. I noticed that Mr. Smith lingered in the waiting room, rather than brave the cold; the temperature outside was down to ten degrees and snow was falling. I saw some familiar faces in the crowd: the Goddess of the Night holding a tray of cookies; Caleb was there, staring down as he drew on a large pad; Derek, without any Tribbles I hoped; Vince and others. The pile of gifts under our little tree was bigger. The coffee maker from the break room was on the counter, along with some cider. Miss James stood beside me.

"Here's Curley's EKG. Looks like he's had an old MI, nothing acute," she reported.

I glanced at the cardiogram and agreed with her assessment.

"No one has registered. I guess they just wanted a party and a place to get away from the cold."

"...Shall I play for him? Par rum pa pa pum. On my drum..."

"I like Curley's choice of music," I commented. "None of this politically correct 'seasonal' music that leaves out the true meaning of Christmas."

I stood and listened, but then I heard something odd.

"HOLD IT," I shouted. "Stop for a minute!"

Silence filled the air, except for one distinct sound, a baby's cries. I stood up on a chair and saw it, a large shoebox, just inside the door, clearly illuminated by the light at the entrance. I ran to it and picked it up.

Sure enough, carefully wrapped inside was a baby, a very small baby. I carried the child towards the back and handed it to Miss James.

"Keep them going," I whispered to Curley. And I left to go examine our new young patient.

It was a baby boy, maybe only a few hours old, but healthy. And, he sure had good lungs, crying the entire time I was listening and palpating. He had been wrapped in a thin blanket and an old worn jacket had been stuffed into his makeshift cradle. His diaper was a soiled handkerchief.

We'd received abandoned babies before; usually they were accompanied by a note, which would read something like this: "I'm sorry, but I can't take care of Walter (or Judy or fill in the blank). Please help him find a good home."

"I'll call him John," I announced. "He is a John Doe, at least for now. We need to call CPS."

Miss James winced at those three letters. She hated turning children, especially babies, over to the system to be shunted from foster home to foster home and, far too often, finishing their childhood on the streets or worse.

"Who's on for them today?" I asked.

"Just our luck, it's Jody. Poor John will be here for a while, especially on Christmas Eve."

Miss James dutifully made the call to CPS, not expecting a return call for several hours. Jody was a caseworker who took the expression methodical to its zenith.

We fixed John up with a proper diaper and wrapped him in a clean blanket and gave him a bottle filled with proper newborn formula.

"Looks like a beautiful, healthy boy. Just look at those eyes and so much black hair," Miss James observed.

"He is a good looking boy, that's for sure. I've never seen a newborn that was so alert; look at him staring at me, sizing me up. He's got a bit of a dark complexion. Maybe he's of Mediterranean origin. Well, no matter. Let's go back to the celebration."

We put young John in a proper cradle, one of our clear plastic bassinettes, and carried him out to the lobby. Curley and Cupcake were keeping the party rolling along with a few jokes.

"What's the difference between a Jew and a canoe?"
"I don't know, what is the difference?"
"One tips."

"Two stupid guys want to go bear hunting, so they ask the Ranger where they can find the bears. He answers 'that's easy, just follow the signs.'

"So they drive along and see a sign which says 'Hunting, Bear Left.' So they turned around and went home."

"Maybe, we better stick to singing," Curley remarked and they started in on a new song.

"Joy to the World, the Lord is come. Let Earth receive her King…"

As the singing started Cupcake whispered something into Miss James ear and the two left together. I was curious, but stayed behind, keeping one eye on the baby who was now safely tucked away in his clear cradle sitting in front of the reception desk. After a few minutes Miss James returned.

"Can you come look at Cupcake," she whispered in my ear.

I left the party and followed Miss James back to Room One where Cupcake was on the exam table wearing one of our paper gowns.

"I noticed it about a month ago. I didn't want to worry Curley, but it's gotten bigger. It doesn't hurt."

"What is it?" I asked.

"She has a lump under her right arm," Miss James reported.

"No fever or pain?" I asked.

"No, it's nothing I'm sure," Cupcake decided. "Just forget about it."

"No, you're here. I might as well check it."

I probed under her arm and immediately felt a golf ball size mass, which was mobile, nontender. I palpated above her clavicle and felt several more lumps, all hard and slightly irregular.

"Lay back and put your arm up over your head," I instructed.

I began examining her right breast and felt the mass at 10:00, about two and a half centimeters, hard, irregular, almost certainly a cancer.

"I'm sorry, Cupcake, but this is almost certainly a breast cancer. Of course a biopsy needs to be done, but I'm 99% sure. We can refer you to one of the surgeons to do the biopsy and then you should see Dr. Bakemyer, a very good and compassionate Oncologist."

She stared down at the floor and then jumped off the table and started to get dressed.

"Don't tell Curley. It's Christmas and our anniversary. I don't want to spoil it for him."

"Don't you think he would want to know?" Miss James asked.

"He probably knows already, just won't admit it. What we said before is not far from the truth. I know I shouldn't say this, but sex just gets better and better even when you're no longer spring chickens. When you're young it's all hurry up and then what? When you get older you can take the time to be indulgent, and after sixty five years we don't have any secrets. You two should remember that. Now, let's go back to the party."

The lobby was full as Curley stood on a table, leading the way with a vigorous rendition of "Angels We Have Heard On High." And then "Hark the Herald."

He looked a bit sweaty to me, but he still had his ever present smile. Cupcake climbed up on the table next to him and took his hand in hers. He turned to her, smiled his special smile, and then he collapsed, falling forward into her arms. The two of them fell from the table, their fall broken by myself and Miss James.

"LOOK AT CURLEY," Cupcake screamed as tears welled up in her eyes.

Curley was ashen gray and was not breathing. I put my fingers on his neck and did not feel a pulse.

"CRASH CART," I yelled to Miss James but she was ahead of me, wheeling the red cart out as I lay Curley flat on the floor and pounded on his chest.

"SOMEONE CALL 911, PLEASE," I shouted, hoping one of the revelers would respond.

We took a quick look with the monitor and saw V. Fib. We prepared to shock him as Miss James manned the ambu bag.

"EVERYBODY CLEAR?" I asked/screamed as I pushed the buttons and Curley jerked off the floor. With that shock, the lights went out. Our monitor still reported V. Fib as the emergency lights came on and a few of our shocked onlookers lit candles.

I warmed up the paddles to shock him again. Once more he jerked off the floor. This time he responded with a faint regular blip on the screen. I felt his carotid, but still there was no pulse. We started chest compressions.

"AMBULANCE IS ON THE WAY," I heard someone scream.

All this commotion and noise and not a peep from that baby boy. Very odd.

It's strange the things which go through your mind in moments of crisis. In the midst of all this chaos, I heard the clock chime twelve.

"Give Epi," I ordered. Luckily Curley still had an IV in his arm.

"Already done."

"Bicarb, Calcium."

"Done."

No pulse still. We're going to lose him.

The chiming of the clock stopped and, all of the sudden, the room became eerily quiet, almost like time had stopped momentarily. There was silence and the only lights were the candles and a faint light from baby John's bassinette.

All of a sudden I felt Curley move. He took a big breath. I felt his neck and was rewarded with a strong carotid pulse. Curley sat up and looked around.

"Did I miss some excitement?" he inquired.

I sat back on the floor, wiped the sweat away from my forehead and stared in amazement. Twenty seconds earlier Curley had been prostrate, dying, and now he looked like he was ready to go out dancing with his precious Cupcake. Curley got up from the floor, while I helped Miss James to her feet.

Cupcake came running and put her arms around Curley's neck and showered him with kisses. Then she slapped him on the cheek.

"Don't you ever scare me like that again, you understand?" she scolded.

Curley's look of surprise was replaced by his smile. "Yes dear," was all he could say.

"Open the presents," Vince shouted.

So we celebrated that Christmas with our patients. We had had quite a haul. Two cheap stethoscopes, a chrome urinal, a box of condoms, some candy, "The Complete Kama Sutra," His and Her underwear, and a few other things, which escape my memory.

It was after we opened the presents that the true extent of the Christmas miracle became apparent. I ran another EKG on Curley. It was normal. I don't mean it was back to his baseline. I mean it was cold normal. No sign of previous MI or anything.

Cupcake beckoned for me to follow her back to one of the exam rooms. She pulled up her blouse and asked me to examine her again. To our amazement, the lumps in her breast and under her arm were gone.

Then Rodney Smith stopped me and pulled up his pant leg. His laceration was completely healed. As a matter of fact, it was like it had never happened. No sutures, no scar, nothing.

I wondered how many others who were there were cured of their maladies? Was "the Goddess of the Night" free of her cancer? Were Caleb's headaches gone forever? I didn't bother to ask. It was three a.m. and they all started to file out with many "Merry Christmas's heard in the waiting room and out on the street as they left.

"Thank you, Dr. Barnes, for saving my life," Curley said as he effusively shook my hand once again. I gave him a smile and he smiled back. "Although I wish you really were the Dr. Barnes of "The Institute for Penile Rejuvenation."

"I don't know," I answered. "From what Cupcake said I don't think you need any help in that department."

We all turned red at my comment as they left.

Cupcake turned to us as she walked out the door. "Don't forget about us when it's time for you two to tie the knot."

Finally, everyone was gone.

"What about baby John?" Miss James wondered.

"Where is baby John?" I asked with more than a hint of worry in my voice.

The bassinette was gone and so was John. The phone rang at that moment. It was Jody, finally answering our call.

"Get a number and tell her we'll call her back," I requested as I desperately searched the waiting room.

"You don't think someone took him, do you?" I asked.

Miss James appeared remarkably calm, considering we'd misplaced a newborn baby.

"Maybe this is the answer?" She stated as she held up a drawing, the one Caleb had been frantically working on.

It was a manger scene. There were sheep and cows and Mary and Joseph. Shepherds were at the door and there was Jesus. Only he wasn't in a manger. He was laying in a clear plastic bassinette with the words "Clinic" clearly stenciled on the side.

"It can't be, can it?" I asked.

There were some words at the bottom: "God touches our lives in mysterious and unexpected ways."

The Clinic was empty now. The ambulance finally arrived and we sent it away. We called back Jody and told her "never mind."

I looked at the card Curley had given me.

Curley and Cupcake
Troubadours
Weddings, Bar Mitzvahs, Birthdays
Bachelor and Bachelorette Parties
877-555-0000

"Happy Anniversary," I whispered and I took Miss James' hand.

The snow had stopped and we went outside to a cold, clear night filled with stars. There was a bright star in the distance, which seemed to be moving to the east.

"Merry Christmas, Doctor," she whispered.

"Merry Christmas, Nurse."

NEXT NIGHT CLINIC

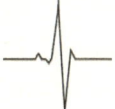

"COME ON, COME ON, CHANGE ALREADY," I YELLED AT THE light. "Finally. Seven Forty? I'll never hear the end of it... Move it up there... Stay green. Finally, there it is... Seven fifty five... I guess that's not too late. And, it's a full moon."

I should never have finished watching that movie; should have left earlier so that I wouldn't be late again. I've already seen it five times. Galaxy Quest*. A stupid movie anyway. "Activate the Omega Thirteen" and go back in time thirteen seconds. What I need is the Omega Ten Thousand.

I tried to sneak in the back, but no luck. Not only was Miss James not there, but the Medical Director was and he did not look happy.

"Sorry, I'm late, Dr. Olsen," I tried to explain, "but I had trouble finishing my shift at the hospital and traffic was bad and I had to feed Jenny..."

Dr. Olsen just stood there with his arms folded across his chest. He wore black rimmed glasses, was short, bald, and round, and he wouldn't have known a varicose vein from a hemorrhoid. He was the ultimate pencil pusher; rules and regulations were all he knew.

"Jenny?" he asked in his squeaky, nasal, monotone voice.

"My dog, a mutt, part terrier, part collie, and a lot of parts we aren't sure of," I explained trying to lighten the mood.

"Stop, Dr. Barnes," he held up his hand and shook his head. Beads of sweat landed on my scrubs. "I don't care about Jenny. I don't care about your other job. I don't want any excuses. You've been warned repeatedly, we've even overlooked a few minutes here and there because you're a good doctor, but fifty eight minutes is unacceptable. It's my job to see that this Clinic is properly staffed; twenty four hours a day, seven days a week, without interruption. I'm afraid that after tonight your services will no longer be needed here. Good evening."

That was it. He walked out. No discussion, no appeal, nothing.

"That was rough, Dr. Barnes," the nurse tried to console me. "I'm Judy, Judy Small. I usually work L&D, so I'll need a little guidance. All the rooms are full. Fifteen-year-old with belly pain is in One; eighteen-year-old girl with a laceration of the arm in Two, some sort of altercation I think; a patient with a headache in Three; and swollen legs in Four."

Just great. A rookie nurse, all the rooms full already, and I'm out of a job. I knew I should have stayed in bed today.

I picked up the chart to One. Jeremiah Baker, fifteen, no medical problems, lower abdominal pain for two days. No fever, vitals normal. At least he should be fairly straightforward.

I knocked and opened the door.

"Good evening, Jeremiah. I'm Dr. Barnes. What is the problem you are having?"

"Hi, Dr. Barnes," he greeted me with an enthusiastic handshake. "Jeremiah. I'm really happy to meet you."

He flashed a huge, wide grin and then winced slightly, as he held his right side. I wasn't a surgeon, but I already was making a diagnosis of appendicitis.

"What's the problem you're having?" I asked again.

"I've got this pain in my abdomen, right here," and he pointed to McBurney's point. "It started yesterday and just won't go away."

"Any nausea or vomiting or fever?" I continued, taking his history.

"I threw up once last night and I haven't eaten anything all day. It's appendicitis, isn't it, Dr. Barnes. I've got all the symptoms, don't I?" and he flashed his grin again.

"So far I'd say you're batting a thousand. Lay down here and let me check your abdomen," I requested.

Jeremiah lay on the exam table as I gently palpated and percussed his abdomen. When I reached his right lower quadrant, he visibly winced and the localized rigidity was classic peritonitis.

"Well, young man," I began, "you almost certainly have acute appendicitis. I'm sure you'll need an appendectomy, but we don't do surgery here. I'm going to call Dr. Forstey at University Hospital and get you on his service. He's a great surgeon and he'll take good care of you. In the meantime, we'll start an IV and give you some antibiotics and make the arrangements to get you to the hospital. Are your parents around?"

"My mom was here, but she had to go to work and left about five minutes before you came in, but I'll call her," Jeremiah said.

Then he added, "You know Dr. Barnes, I knew it was appendicitis. I did some reading and I knew I had all the classic symptoms. And, I've been studying really hard, because I'm going to be a doctor, like you. There are a lot of bad things that go on in this neighborhood, gangs, drugs, lots of crime, but most of the kids, they know about you. They know that you come here from the University and that you care. That's the kind of doctor I'll be; one who cares."

He gave me one of his big smiles and I smiled back.

"Thanks for the compliment, Jeremiah," I replied. "Just lie here and the nurse will be in in a few minutes."

I scribbled some orders on his chart and called Nurse Small and told her to start an IV and begin Jeremiah on IV Zosyn. Then I called Zack Forstey and arranged for transfer to University Hospital. I moved on to Room Two and the lacerated arm.

I glanced at the chart for Kelly Montague, eighteen, laceration of the left arm. No medical problems, no allergies...

Hmm, did that boy with appendicitis have any allergies? I don't remember what the chart said.

I went back to Room One and looked for Jeremiah's chart.

The nurse must have it in the back.

I stuck my head in the room.

"Do you have any allergies?" I inquired. I saw Nurse Small hanging the IV fluids and the medication. One thing about those L&D nurses: they were really good at starting IV's. I still did not see his chart.

"Not that I know of, Dr. Barnes," Jeremiah answered. "Do you want me to check with my mom?"

I thought for a moment.

He's fifteen; he should know.

"That's OK. I'll be back in a few minutes and the ambulance is on the way."

I went back to the lacerated arm.

"Good evening, Miss Montague. How did you cut your arm?" I started what I hoped would be a short interview.

"I did it, Doctor, I cut it. I wanted to kill myself. That'll show that Gerald. He'll miss me when I'm gone, that miserable creep," she ranted.

Just what I need, a hysterical, suicidal teenager.

"Calm down, Miss Montague. I'm sorry about Gerald. I'm sure he is the biggest creep in the world, but I need to know about your arm."

"How dare you call my man a creep. Who do you think you are, Mister Dr. Bigshot? Gerald is ten times the man you are. I'm not staying here and letting you insult him and me. Good-bye, Doctor Bigshot."

And she stormed out of the Clinic. Oh well, you win some and you lose some.

I made a note on her chart: "Left AMA, did not sign the form," and went on to the next patient, Elias Trowbridge, fifty three, with a headache for twelve hours.

I started to knock on the door when I felt a grab on my sleeve.

"Come to Room One, something's terribly wrong," Nurse Small shouted. She was white as a sheet and her hand was shaking.

I raced back to One and found Jeremiah on the table, IV in his arm, he was blue from head to toe, convulsing and not breathing.

"What happened?" I screamed as I picked up the ambu bag and tried to ventilate him. I vainly felt for a pulse. "Get the crash cart and give me some Epi."

I saw the bag of antibiotics hanging, half of it infused and strongly suspected anaphylactic shock.

"Epi, open up the IV, start chest compressions," I commanded.

Nurse Small dutifully obeyed as I picked up the laryngoscope.

"All I see is a big swollen tongue. I can't get passed it. Get me a scalpel."

I'd never done an emergency trach or cricothyrotomy on a live person, only on a dummy, but I had seen my surgical colleagues do them. I saw no alternative at that moment.

I splashed some Betadine on Jeremiah's neck, felt for the appropriate landmarks and started to cut.

There's a first time for everything.

After an eternity of slicing through skin and fat and I'm not sure what else, I entered the airway. After a few missteps I managed to slide a size 6 ET tube in and stared to ventilate Jeremiah. I had been at it for a total of twelve minutes, but it seemed like twelve hours. Jeremiah wasn't responding, however. No effort to breath, no pulse and the EKG was flat.

"Start CPR," we said simultaneously. But, it was futile. He was gone.

Now what? Call Mrs. Baker and tell her, 'Good evening, I'm sorry to inform you your son is dead.' This night has gone from bad to worse.

"Dr. Barnes?"

"Yes, Miss Small."

"I'm sorry. I don't know what happened. I started the Zosyn and then, all of a sudden, he turned blue, he stopped breathing and started seizing. Was it something I did?"

I looked at her face. Tears were streaming down both cheeks.

"No, nurse. It was what I did."

Why is it always people like Jeremiah? Why do good people have to die? Why? Why?

Where is his chart, anyway?

I left to go back to the break room, closed the door, sat down, and stared at my hands.

"Dr. Barnes, please come to Room Two," Miss Small's voice sounded over the intercom.

I shook myself free from my moment of anguish and trudged down the hall towards Exam Room Two. I heard a woman scream.

"What's going on in...?" I started to ask as I bulled my way into the room. My question was immediately answered by the sight of a young woman, maybe fifteen years old, up in stirrups, obviously in labor. Miss Small was checking her as I walked in.

"She's ten and ready to push, Dr. Barnes," Miss Small reported.

I hate delivering babies.

"It says she arrived two hours ago. Why didn't she transfer to the hospital?"

"With all the excitement, I guess she feel through the cracks," Miss Small answered.

I glanced at her name, Barbi Genter, then I donned a gown and gloves and went to work.

"OK, Miss Genter, when I tell you to push, you push, like you're trying to send this baby across the room. When I tell you to breathe, you should take quick, deep breaths until I tell you to push again, OK?"

She grunted, which I took as an affirmative. I could see dark hair and then the head was all the way down.

"Easy, no Barbi, wait for the next contraction and we'll have this baby out in no time."

I was hoping to get the kid out without an episiotomy. I had my hand on the baby's head when my patient gave a hard push and the head popped out followed by the rest of a healthy looking baby girl, which was followed by a large amount of blood from some-where. I quickly passed the baby off and then went to work trying to find the source of what was a lot of bright red blood.

"Check the baby fast, Miss Small. I'm going to need some help here. Oh, and turn on that Pitocin."

Maybe that will help.

No such luck. Blood was pouring out and I was feeling helpless to stop it. I reached my hand up inside and felt the disrupted uterus and then I picked up the sheet, which lay across Barbi's abdomen, and saw the low transverse scar.

"How many C-Sections have you had before, Miss Benton?"

There was no answer as I glanced at the monitor, which revealed a heart rate of 140 and BP of 60.

"Open up the IV and call an ambulance, Miss Small," I screamed as calmly as I could, as I quickly delivered a torn placenta. The bleeding didn't stop, however. I started to pack sponge after sponge into the uterus and vagina and then watched as her abdomen started to get bigger and her blood pressure and then her pulse started to sink even lower.

"Epi, Bicarb, Calcium, the kitchen sink," I ordered.

The ambulance arrived, finally. She was alive, but barely. She had a heart rate of 120 and BP of 70 as they packed her into the ambulance and sped away, both mother and baby.

How many more hours until seven?

There was a woman waiting for me as I walked out of Room Two.

"Dr. Barnes?" she asked.

"Yes?"

"I'm Dorothy Baker. I got a call about my son? The lady told me it was urgent."

I'm not ready for this.

"Wait for me in Room Three. I'll be with you in a moment," I said, trying to calm my trembling voice.

"Is Jeremiah OK? Please tell me."

I stepped into the room with her. I'm sure she sensed that something was terribly wrong.

"Jeremiah is dead," I reported to her, far too matter-of-factly, I decided, too late. "We were sure he had appendicitis and we were getting him ready to go the hospital, he was given IV fluids and antibiotics, and then he suddenly arrested and I couldn't save him."

She looked at me funny for a moment, then put her hand to her mouth and her eyes became wide, as she began to fathom the true meaning of my words.

"NOOOOO, NOT MY BABY," she screamed and she pounded on my chest. "Antibiotics? You gave him Penicillin, didn't you? He almost died when he was two from a dose of Penicillin."

I took a step back and almost passed out, collapsing into the chair.

"I asked him if he had any allergies and he said no," I muttered.

"I WROTE IT ON THE FORM, IT WAS THERE IN BLACK AND WHITE, YOU... YOU KILLED MY BABY," she screamed and then she slapped my face and walked out.

I'm sure it said NKDA, or did it? Did I even look at the history?

I felt my medical career slipping away from me as I jumped up and ran to check Jeremiah's medical history. The chart had magically appeared at the nurse's station. She was right. Allergy: Penicillin.

How could I miss that? How can I keep being a doctor when something like this has happened?

Miss Small came in at that moment, ashen, tears streaming down her face.

"How could we both overlook something like that?" she asked, not expecting an answer. She sat next to me, neither one of us knowing what to say.

"There's only one more patient here, everyone else has left," she finally remarked. "Maybe you can see her real quick and then we'll close the Clinic for the last hour."

I turned and looked at her, nodded my head, and managed to drag myself down the hall to Room Four. There was a smell emanating from beneath the door, a familiar scent of dried sweat, unwashed clothes, and decaying life which was common among the many homeless individuals who came to the Clinic for medical care, warmth, and the occasional handout. I glanced at the name, Gladys Wentworth, "Gussie" to those of us familiar with the neighborhood population.

"CC: Swollen legs…"

"Hello Gussie, legs still bothering you?" I asked, obviously barely interested in her answer.

"The demons are out tonight," she whispered. "They're all over; saw a nasty one right outside. Full moon. No one's safe. Here take this, quick. It'll keep them away."

She handed me a garland of dried apricots and prunes.

"Put it on," she commanded.

I complied just to speed things along.

Gussie was about five foot nothing, weighed about three hundred pounds, despite having only two teeth. She always wore a heavy coat over seven or eight layers of clothes, even if it was a hundred degrees. Her skin was wrinkled and grimy and she was accompanied by a small cart which contained all her worldly possessions. She was diagnosed with schizophrenia; her state of cognition dependent on whether she had remembered to take her medication. And, she was plagued by chronically swollen legs which brought her into the Clinic on a regular basis.

"You taking your meds, Gussie?" I asked as I started to look at her legs.

"Twice a day, without fail," she answered. "If I didn't I'd be seeing things and hearing voices."

"But there are demons out tonight?" I inquired. Normally I ignored her commentary, limiting my work to treating her legs. However, with all that had happened this night, I was grasping at any explanation for the series of disasters.

"Terrible demons. The devil's workers. That necklace will keep them away," she whispered in my ear. "If you still see them, add a few cloves of garlic and for sure they'll leave you be."

Her legs weren't as bad as usual. Discolored and edematous, but no ulcers or signs of infection.

"Keep doing what…" I started, but she interrupted me.

"This is the last one. I stole it from Aladdin. His last wish. He thinks it's in that lamp, but I took the wish and now it's mine. I just can't decide how to use it."

She held up a small glass jar with a cork in the top.

"It's just an empty bottle," I said, being in no mood to humor her. I was growing tired of our encounter and just wanted her to be gone.

"Just elevate your legs as much as possible, Gussie, and you'll be OK. I see that you're supposed to be seen at the hospital next week. Please keep that appointment."

"But, Dr. Barnes… the demons, what about them?"

I looked at her eyes, which were looking around wildly and I took the garland from around my neck.

"Here, Gussie. You wear mine, too. That way you'll be twice as protected."

She smiled at me and took the wreath of fruit and gleefully put it on.

"You're all set now," I reassured her.

"Thank you, Doctor, thank you," she said effusively and she shook my hand.

I saw Jeremiah in that handshake and pulled my hand away.

"You're OK, Gussie, but please leave," I muttered as I opened the door.

She looked at my face, her eyes betraying a look of fear, but not fear of unseen demons, it was fear of me, as if I was the demon. She wheeled her cart out the door and disappeared into the early morning. The sun was starting to rise and there was light fog. It was six forty five.

Fifteen minutes left in my medical career.

Back at my apartment I lay down reflecting on the night's events, mulling everything over and over, but always coming back to the smiling face of Jeremiah and the unseen words written on his chart: ALLERGY: PENICILLIN. ALLERGY: PENICILLIN. ALLER…

Of course it wasn't the first time I'd made a mistake; residency is an endless stream of "learning experiences" as Dr. Gottlieb liked to call them. But, there is a difference between mistakes in judgment and carelessness. It was a difference I didn't think I could live with.

I lay back on my couch and knocked my white coat to the floor and heard a loud "Thud."

What's that?

I picked up the coat and felt something in the pocket, an empty jar, crazy Gussie's wish in a bottle. I stared at the empty jar and looked at it from every angle. It was just an empty jar.

Hmm… no, she's loony. Still, it can't hurt to try. Now what were the Genie in Aladdin's rules? 1. Can't kill anyone; 2. Can't bring people back from the dead; and 3. Can't make anyone fall in love with someone else. I don't need one or three. But number two is a problem. Maybe there's a way around it…

"What am I thinking? It's just an empty jar. Gussie's crazy. Besides, Jeremiah's dead," I concluded out loud. "Maybe if I…"

I took the cork out and closed my eyes.

"Nothing."

I put the cork back in the jar, tossed it in the garbage and lay down on the couch, trying to decide if I should become a dishwasher or a waiter.

Maybe I'll end up in jail.

Hours later I was awakened by the phone ringing.

"Hello," I answered, sleep still in my voice.

"Don't tell me you're sleeping. Get your ass up and get to the Clinic," Miss James commanded. "You can't be late again. Edith told me that Olsen is going to be there and that if you're late one more time, you'll be fired."

"Uh, Ok, but I was already fi…" I started to say, but then I stopped myself. "Hold on just a second."

I looked at my phone. It was yesterday and I had an hour to make it to the Clinic. I looked in the garbage, no empty jar.

"Thanks for calling me, my sweet wonderful nurse. I'm on my

way."

I jumped into a new set of scrubs and hopped in my car. I hit every light on the way and made it to the Clinic twenty minutes early. Dr. Olsen saw me, said "Good Evening," and left.

Jeremiah was there with his mother, was diagnosed with appendicitis, and started on Levaquin. He was transferred to the hospital for an uneventful appendectomy. Kelly Montague had her arm sewed up and was released to Psych. Barbi Genter showed up in labor and was transferred to the hospital before she had progressed too far.

Finally there was only one more patient to be seen, a homeless woman with swollen legs, Gussie.

"Good evening, Gussie, what's the problem you've been having? Your legs again?" I started my usual speech, trying to hide the excitement in my voice.

"It's a good night to be out. No monsters or demons. The streets are safe from evil spirits," she announced.

"I agree with you, Gussie. Now, let me take a look at your legs."

Her legs showed their usual swelling and changes of venous stasis. I admonished her to wear her support stockings and keep her legs elevated and to keep her appointments at the hospital clinic. As she was getting ready to leave I saw the empty glass jar.

"A wish?" I asked her pointing to the jar.

"A wish? Nope, just a glass jar I found in a dumpster over on Maple," she said in her mumbling voice. But, she looked at me and smiled as she gathered her cart and belongings and left.

I smiled back.

True second chances should be cherished. They are a rare and precious gift.

In the movie Galaxy Quest, *the Omega Thirteen is a device which, when activated, allows an individual to relive the last thirteen seconds of his or her life.*

Night Clinic Superheros

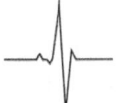

"COLD, WET, AND DREARY," I MUTTERED, SHAKING THE water off my coat. "It should make for a quiet night."

"Now you've jinxed us," Miss James remarked as she patted me on my butt. "But, then again, nobody's here at the moment, so maybe you'll be right, for a change."

She looked at me and then at the clock.

"Ten minutes early. Maybe miracles can happen," she commented.

I just smiled as we took the time for a cup of coffee while waiting for some business. It wasn't long before the buzz of the front door opening filled our little break room and Miss James went to see our first patient.

"Abdominal pain for four days," she announced when she returned. "I put him in Room One and drew some labs. He doesn't look too sick to me."

"David Rampart, 45... no previous surgery, no allergies... heart rate 65, BP 122/60, no fever..." I read. I knocked on the door and went in.

Mr. Rampart was sprawled out on the exam table, his face flushed with beads of sweat dripping off his forehead.

"Good evening, Mr. Rampart," I began. "What brings you in..."

He turned his head and vomited at my feet before I could finish my usual intro. Luckily, his emesis missed me completely.

Maybe a good omen.

"I've got this terrible pain right here," he reported as he pointed to his right upper abdomen. "It's been going on for two days. I can't eat, nothing makes it go away. My back hurts and I've thrown up about twenty times."

"Ever have a pain like this before?" I asked.

"Never this bad," he answered as he winced in pain.

"Had much to drink recently?"

"Just the usual. No alcohol, just beer. I never touch alcohol."

"How much beer have you had today?" I continued my inquiry.

"Just my usual amount, maybe a twelve pack."

"And how many yesterday?"

"About the same. I drink that amount every day, after I get home from work. But, it's just beer."

I felt his abdomen which was soft, but diffusely tender. There was no scleral icterus. Heart and lungs were normal.

"What kind of work do you do?"

"Cop. I walk the day time beat over on Main and Maple."

"Ever have pancreatitis?"

"Pancrea... what?"

"Inflammation in your pancreas. It can be caused by alcohol and I suspect that is what you have. We'll need to get you to the hospital. And, you should think about giving up drinking beer. It's going to kill you."

He lay on the table with a confused look on his face when Miss James came in.

"Don't tell me," I said, before she had a chance to speak. "His Lipase and amylase are elevated."

"Correct, Dr. Barnes," she responded. "You're some kind of Svengali or something."

She had a big smile on her face and then she added, "Dr. Svengali, I've already called for an ambulance. I'll start an IV and you can go use your amazing talents on a kid with a sore throat in Room Two."

"Thank you, kind Nurse, I will do just that."

I went on to Room Two and quickly dispatched a three-year-old girl with a simple case of Strep throat. The ambulance arrived and

Mr. Rampart was shipped off to the County Hospital.

Business was slow and we had about an hour without any patients. Miss James took out her knitting and worked on a sweater she had started more than a year ago. I took the time to study up on the latest treatments for Non Hodgkin's lymphoma; I was on my last rotation through the Oncology service. Only a few more months and I'd be a finished doctor, almost.

We were both roused by a crash which came from the lobby, followed by the buzz of a patient waiting at the front desk.

We went to investigate and found a portly man dressed in brown tights, with a black and brown striped cape. There was a large "R" embroidered on his chest and on the cape. He wore a black mask which made him look, pardon the pun, bug-eyed. His suit was torn at the right shoulder where there was a deep bloody wound.

"Can I get some help here?" he demanded. "Patch me up quick, I need to get after them before they escape."

"That's a nasty wound you've got there, Mister…?" Miss James observed.

"Roachman, at your service," he replied.

Miss James almost gagged as she tried to stifle her laughter and then she coughed.

"People always seem to get choked up like that when they first see me," Roachman commented.

Miss James composed herself and then handed our patient a clipboard while ushering him into Room Three. She emerged a few minutes later.

"He's got about an eight centimeter laceration on his right shoulder, clean, looks like it was made by a sharp blade; doesn't go into muscle. You should be able to suture it here. We made need to get Psych involved here. Surely he's delusional and may be a danger, if not to others, then to himself."

Just great. A wacko with delusions of grandeur. First things first; check out his wound.

I knocked on the door and went in.

"Good evening, Roachman, I'm Dr. Barnes. Let me check out that shoulder of yours."

I saw him sitting on the exam table, his legs folded. He was licking his hands and then his feet. I noticed an unusual odor and his cape was folded in a funny way, like wings tucked into each other.

"Hello, Dr. Barnes. I'm glad to meet you."

He grabbed my hand and gave it a vigorous shake, leaving a slimy feeling on my hand. I went to the sink and washed my hands and put on some gloves.

"You're the second superhero I've had the privilege of meeting. Captain Surgery popped in here a few months ago and saved the lives of a couple of kids. Anyway, let me look at your shoulder. How'd this happen?"

"Careful, Doctor," he winced as I took the dressing off his shoulder and then he recounted his story. "I came upon an old lady being mugged by some young punks. Of course I had to intervene and that's when I got this. Believe me, those two punks got much worse. They're probably in Intensive Care."

"I'll get this stitched up in no time, go on, tell me about Roach-man."

I cleaned the wound with some chlorhexidine and injected some local anesthetic as he began his story.

"Well, Dr. Barnes, I'm sure you've heard of Spiderman and Batman and the Wolverine, all with their special powers. But what's so great about spiders or bats? What do spiders do? Spin a web, crawl around, wait for some poor unsuspecting fly to fall into their trap? Big deal. Bats are even more mundane. They can fly, so? Batman is all hype. A fancy car, fancy toys and attitude. And Spiderman? He's more screwed up than most of the villains he faces. Guilt should not be part of the superhero gestalt. Ow..."

"Sorry, I guess I didn't numb that spot. Go on."

"But roaches, there's something timeless and almost invincible about us. No matter how hard you try to get rid of us, we just keep being around. And, if there's a nuclear apocalypse or some other natural disaster, if the earth gets smashed out of its orbit around the sun by an asteroid, who do you think will survive? I'd bet on us; the roaches and the rats."

"First layer is done. Now just the skin to close. What about roaches and rats?"

"We're survivors, that's all. A million years from now, when humans have been wiped away from the face of this planet, the rats and roaches will survive."

"I guess that's good news for my Uncle Sacha," I observed.

Roachman gave me a dirty look and then continued his story.

"I discovered my special powers about a year ago. I was working at the waste collection center, shoveling garbage into the furnaces and compactors. So, one day I slip and fall into the trash compactor. I did all I could to avoid its vicious grinders and wheels, but needless to say I was mangled to the point where I was almost dead. It was a Friday and that Monday was a holiday, so I would have been left for days if it hadn't been for them."

"Them?" I asked, almost afraid of what the answer would be.

"The roaches. One roach alone can only do so much. But, put a hundred thousand together and they become quite formidable. They managed to carry me out of there and nursed me back to health. It took months, but I survived and with a new appreciation for my saviors. But, even more amazing, as I healed I felt something new, a power flowing though my veins. I had super powers, Roach powers, and I vowed to use them for good; to restore the good name of the cockroach forever."

I finished putting a dressing on his shoulder.

He seems crazy and he may be a danger to himself. We'd better have him evaluated at the hospital.

"Uh... Roachman, wait here for a few minutes. I want to check your shoulder before you leave," I instructed.

I left him alone and went to find Miss James.

"I've already called the hospital," she reported. "They're sending an ambulance. Oh, and there's another patient in Room One. You might be interested in this one. He claims he was attacked by a rat wearing a cape."

"First roaches and now rats. What's going on here?" I asked no one in particular.

I picked up the chart outside Room One. Manuel Custer, 28, no medical problems, complaining of "rat bite."

"Good Evening, Mr. Custer, I'm Dr. Barnes. What's the problem that brought you in here tonight?" I greeted him, with my usual bedside banter.

"Man, Dr. Barnes, it was a rat, big as a German Shepherd, attacked me and bit me right here."

He pointed to his arm where there was an ugly wound, macerated, but not bleeding.

"What time did this happen?"

"About an hour ago. I was just minding my own business, walking down the street. First I feel something crawl up my leg."

"The huge rat?" I asked.

"No… no, it was a roach. Crawled right along my chest and between my eyes. Well, I swatted it away and then there was this rat, wearing a black cape, stood up on its hind legs and took a bite out of my arm. Well, I pulled out my knife and took a swipe at it. Then, this fat guy in tights and a mask shows up and I get him instead. That fat guy had a cape on, too. Well, it was just too weird for me, so I got out of there. I'm telling you this neighborhood ain't safe. Vicious roaches, giant rats, and crazy fat dudes."

I was beginning to think that maybe Roachman wasn't so crazy, but then a thought crossed my head. First I dressed Mr. Custer's wound and applied some topical local anesthetic. Then I went back to Room Three.

"Let me check this wound before you go," I requested as I peaked at Roachman's bandage, which was dry.

"By the way," I continued, "does Roachman have a sidekick? Batman has Robin and the Green Hornet has Kato or something."

"Well, yes, as a matter of fact, I do. He's right here. Super Rat."

He reached under his cape and pulled out a medium-sized rat with gray brown fur and wearing a black cape with a large "R" on it. Roachman held his companion up and then kissed the rat on its nose.

"He's the best, most reliable buddy anyone could have. He saved me from those muggers tonight."

Curioser and curioser.

"What did Super Rat do, if I might be so bold to ask?" I inquired.

"Why, he drove them off. Bit one of them on the arm, he did. Those cowards took off as if they'd seen a ghost."

"Was one of the muggers about five-foot-ten, black curly hair, thick black moustache, really thin?"

"Yeah, how'd you know?"

"Let's just say that we doctors have some super powers also. Wait here for a few more minutes, please, and we might catch one of the muggers."

"They're here, the muggers, I knew it, I felt it. One thing about us roaches and rats: we have an uncanny ability to sense when garbage is nearby. Let us at 'em. We'll teach them to leave poor defenseless ladies alone."

"You just wait here while I call the police. I don't want you getting cut any worse."

"No mugger scares me. I'm Roachman and I can vanquish the vilest villains this world can dish out."

"I'm sure you can, but you've done your part for tonight. It's time to let the police do their job."

As I left him, Miss James grabbed me and whispered in my ear, "I think another of the muggers is in Room Four."

"Call the police, Nurse, while I check out our new patient."

She nodded as I picked up the chart outside Room Four.

Malcolm Johnson, twenty-two, no medical problems, chief complaint, insect bites on the groin, rat bite on leg.

"Good evening, Mr. Johnson, I'm Dr. Barnes. From your chart it looks like you have been attacked while visiting a garbage dump or sewer. What happened?"

"I don't know, exactly. I was minding my own business when this huge roach crawled up my leg and bit me. It took me a while to shoe it away and then this big rat comes out of nowhere and bites me, right through my jeans. I'm not going to get the plague, am I? I hear that rats carry the plague."

"We'll just have to wait and see, won't we," I replied as I scribbled some notes on his chart.

"Tell me, Mr. Johnson, why do you think a roach and a rat would attack you? What were you doing? And, did you see where they went? We might need to try to catch that rat and have it tested, to see if it's carrying the Plague. In the meantime, let me check your injuries."

I handed him a gown and told him I'd be back in few minutes. I found Miss James in the front.

"Mr. Custer and Mr. Johnson definitely have some bond between them. They each have a dragon tattooed on their left forearm," I reported.

"The police are on the way, as a matter of fact, there they are now," Miss James answered as we both noticed the flashing lights outside. We greeted two uniformed officers at the door when we all heard it:

"YEOW, GET AWAY, GET AWAY."

We hurried to Room Four and found Mr. Johnson cowering in the corner, looking like he had been accosted by the devil himself. I heard some scurrying from somewhere in the room, but I didn't see anyone or anything. Then there was a second scream from down the hall. One of the officers and Miss James stayed with the terrified Mr. Johnson while I took the other policeman to investigate Mr. Custer.

"There he goes… look there," Mr. Custer said with terror in his voice, pointing to the far corner of the room.

"I don't see any..." Officer Krupa started to say, but then we both saw him or it. A big, dark brown roach, the size of a big mouse. It raced under a table and when we pulled that table away from the wall, it was gone.

"Stay here, Officer," I requested and I stepped out of Room Four and into Room Three where I found Roachman calmly sitting in the chair stroking the belly of Super Rat.

"Sorry, Roachman, but there's been some excitement. You haven't left this room?"

"Not for a moment, Dr. Barnes," and he licked his hands again before resuming his gentle caressing of Super Rat.

I don't know why I find Roachman so disgusting... Yes, I do know why.

I went back to Room Four.

"What did you see, Mr. Custer?" I queried.

"It was a roach, eight feet tall, standing over me, threatening me. It threatened to bite my head off, only it wasn't really talking. I mean I heard this voice inside my head and I knew it was from that monster standing over me. There it is again... that voice... AIEEEE!!!"

And he passed out.

Very Kafkaesque.

I turned and saw Roachman in the doorway.

"It's strange what games guilt can play with the mind and soul," he commented and then went back to Room Three.

I went back to Mr. Custer, who was coming around.

"Where am..." he started to say, and then he looked at me and Officer Krupa and blurted out, "I did it, I attacked that lady and stole her purse and beat her up. Please, please, take me away from here. Protect me from them."

"Well, Officer, you can't get a cleaner confession than that, spontaneous, no coercion. Let me finish cleaning up his wounds and then you can have him; rather, both of them. Mr. Johnson was your partner in crime, Mr. Custer?"

"Yes, yes, just get me out of here. I'll feel safer in jail."

The policeman gathered the two petty thieves together in handcuffs and carted them away to jail. I went back to check on our "superheroes."

Room Three was empty. I went out to the lobby just in time to see a large rat with a cape out on the sidewalk. Perched on the back of its neck was a big dark brown roach. I watched in amazement as the rat spread its four legs out and took off, flying through the air with, pardon my English, the greatest of ease. As they made their escape, I heard Roachman's voice inside my head.

"Thanks for patching me up, Dr, Barnes, you did a great job. And, never underestimate the powers that we vermin possess. Remember, when the apocalypse comes and most life on this planet is destroyed, it will be the rats and roaches who inherit the earth."

"Doctor... Dr. Barnes," I heard the voice of Miss James and felt her hand rubbing my shoulder. "Are you OK?"

"Yes, Nurse, I am quite well," I answered, but I think I still had a peculiar look on my face.

"You don't look 'quite well.' You look like you've been staring into the eyes of a vicious monster or something."

"It's funny, Miss James. Something which is good can also be terrifying and it's ironic that this terror can be used to combat evil. I guess it's sort of like the pain one feels from a shot. At first, all the recipient feels is the pain of the injection. The good after effect, be it a vaccination which prevents a dreaded disease or the well being which may come from medication; this may not be associated with the pain at all. Maybe Roachman is something like that. Anyway, I don't think he's any sort of a danger. You can call the hospital and cancel the Psych eval."

She gave me a funny look.

"Roachman is just a crazy fat guy in Spandex with a pet rat, Dr. Barnes. See there he goes."

Sure enough, there was Roachman walking past the Clinic, Super Rat gently cradled in his arm. He smiled and winked as he passed by.

Scent of a Night Clinic

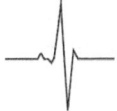

"OH MY GOD, WHAT IS THAT SMELL?" MISS JAMES EX-claimed as I walked into the Clinic. She sniffed me up and down.

"What did you do? Douse yourself with old sweat and then put on a pair of forgotten scrubs from the back of your gym locker?"

"It's not that bad," I responded as she sprayed me down with FOE (Fecal Odor Eliminator).

"It's worse than bad. You'll make our patient's sick just by walking in the room," she commented as she continued to spray. "Why didn't you clean yourself up?"

"Well… I was out running and got back late and I'd forgotten I was scheduled to work tonight and then I only had time to throw on some scrubs and I guess the ones I picked out were already dirty, and here I am."

Miss James smiled and then started to laugh. She sniffed me again.

"A little better, almost tolerable. Hold on a minute; I think I know. I have a solution."

She left me alone and then came back with some clean scrubs; scrubs which were hot pink and almost see through.

"Put these on," she commanded.

"I can't wear these," I protested.

"Well, you can't take care of sick people smelling like a sewer. Come on, at least they're size large. You'll feel much better, I promise and you'll look extra sexy."

She gave me a leering smile and I acquiesced. Actually, I didn't look half bad.

"Pink is definitely my color," I observed as I modeled my new couture for her.

"Enough of the runway show," she stated. "There's a patient in Room One. Diabetic, short of breath."

"Work, work, work, that's all anyone cares about around here. How can a few sick people compare to the world of high fashion," I murmured as I picked up the chart outside the exam room.

"Darrell Preston, 23, diabetic since age ten, takes a lot of insulin," I read.

I opened the door and began my introduction. "Good evening, Mr. Preston, I'm Dr. Barnes. What is the problem that brings you in here?"

He was thin, African American, wearing a hot pink tank top and tight fitting blue jeans. He was sitting on the exam table, no, he was curled up in the corner of the exam table, his arms folded across his legs which were pulled up against his chest. I was greeted by the distinctly fruity scent of ketones.

He looked up at me with a blank stare and groaned.

"Don't say another word, Mr. Preston. I'll be back in a moment."

I stepped out into the hall and started to call for Miss James, but she appeared as if she had read my mind.

"I've already called for an ambulance. I just saw his blood sugar, 585."

"As soon as I walked into the room and noticed the odor, I knew it was DKA; that unmistakable fruity smell. Start an IV of normal saline and run in a liter wide open. Do we have the rest of his BMP?"

"Potassium is 5.3, everything else is normal."

"Get an insulin drip going at one unit per hour, also."

She went to work while I went on to the next patient, Shayla Bakerstreet, abdominal pain, nausea and vomiting for one day, 44, previous hysterectomy. Blood pressure 110/45, heart rate 120.

"Good evening, Miss Bakerstreet. I'm Dr. Barnes. What brought you in here tonight?"

She looked "sick" with flushed cheeks, long, matted brown hair, sunken eyes, and a protuberant belly.

"I'm sick," she announced, stating the obvious. "I started vomiting yesterday, my stomach feels like it's about to explode, I can't go potty; isn't that enough?"

"It is," I replied. I moved a bit closer and the fetid scent of her breath almost drove me back. The typical feculent odor of a small bowel obstruction filled the air.

"How long ago did you have the hysterectomy? And, have you ever had a similar problem before?"

"Ten years ago and no. I've never felt like this, ever," she stated emphatically. "Can't you do something?"

I lightly touched her abdomen and she winced in pain.

"I'm going to throw up," she announced as I started to back away and then moved to help her sit up.

I reached for the basin by the sink and as I gave it to her she vomited, her emesis shooting out several feet and drenching me from chest to knees in vile, sewer-like vomit.

I can't get a break.

"Wait here, Miss Bakerstreet. As you can see I need to see if I can find a change of clothing."

"It's OK, I feel better after throwing up."

I went back to the break room and called for Miss James. She had just finished loading Mr. Preston into the ambulance.

"Oh my god, what happened?" she asked and then she began laughing, uncontrollably, again.

"Yes, yes, very funny. Now is there anything else to wear?"

I had already removed the soiled scrubs and had wrapped a towel around my waist.

"Wait here, I'll see what I can find." And she left.

The TV was blaring as I sat alone in my slightly damp underwear, debating whether to shed them also.

"...Lavender Killer still at large. Victim number eight was discovered today in the posh Evergreen Hills suburb. Similar to the previous seven murders, the victim's throat was cut with almost surgical precision. And, like the other victims, the scent of lavender filled the air at the crime scene. Police have been unable to find any bit of evidence which ties the victims together or demonstrates any sort of pattern…"

Miss James reappeared with a bright purple scrub top and some gray overalls.

"These are all I could find. I don't know if it's a step up from hot pink, but it will have to do."

I eyed my new attire up and down.

"Beggars can't be choosers," I murmured as I pulled the purple scrub shirt over my head, stripped off the dirty underwear, and donned the overalls.

"Let's hope no one looks too closely, Nurse. I don't think this outfit hides everything that is supposed to be hidden. You don't have a belt, do you?"

"I think I have something in my locker, hold on and I'll get I for you."

She returned in a few seconds with a bright yellow belt.

"I think you're ready for the circus, all you need is a big red nose and some floppy shoes," she commented.

"Fun-ny," I remarked. "I'll put on this white coat and I'll be fine."

The coat was a bit small for me. I gazed at my reflection in the mirror: my hair was a bit tousled, the small lab coat made my stomach appear to stick out, I was a kaleidoscope of color in my mismatched outfit. Miss James was correct: I was ready for the circus.

Perhaps my unusual look will bring a bit of lightheartedness to the Clinic.

"There's a sick baby in Room Four, temp 103, diarrhea, runny nose. Could be Rotavirus, there's been a lot of that going around."

"Thank you, Nurse, I guess it's back to work."

I picked up the chart. David Thompson, 3 months old, otherwise healthy. Heart rate 130, temp 103.

"Good evening, I'm Dr. Barnes," I announced. "This is David?"

The woman with him, his mother, I presumed, nodded.

"What's the problem little David is having?"

"He's been coughing and vomiting and his bowels are running and running."

"Is he usually healthy? I mean has he been sick or in the hospital before?"

"Never even been in the hospital. He was born at home and got all his shots at home. He started getting like this yesterday. I gave him some Tylenol, but he's still sick."

"What have you tried to feed him?"

"Why, breast milk, of course; greatest thing God ever made, at least for babies."

"Can't argue with you on that."

I gave her a little smile as I started to examine her child.

"Let me look at your eyes, little David," I whispered. He stared at my face, his eyes wide open. The pupils looked normal and there were tears. I listened to his heart which was racing along at about 130 and his lungs were clear, the only noise was a bit of a rasp from his upper airway which went away after he coughed.

"I'm going to undo his onesie and his diaper now, if that's OK with you," I asked softly.

His abdomen was soft and there was no tenderness. As I started to check his genitalia, he did what all baby boys seemed to like to do to me and peed all over my purple shirt and then on my face as I tried to avoid the yellow stream.

"He should be a fireman," I commented as I wiped urine form my face and chest. "I'm not having much luck with my clothes today. At least it's sterile."

I turned him to inspect his back and he passed a large, green diarrheal stool which ran onto his diaper, the exam table, and onto my shoes.

"Figures," I muttered. "Miss James," I called out, "could you give me some help, please."

In a few moments the door opened and my nurse entered, took one look at me: my purple scrub top was splattered with the spray of urine, there was baby poop on the table, floor, and my shoes, as I held our small patient in one hand and tried to clean up with the other. Miss James did what any conscientious nurse would do in such a situation: she burst out in uncontrollable laughter, for the third time.

"Dr. Barnes, you really should take greater care to control your bodily functions," she remarked as she took our young patient from my hands and handed him back to his mother, who immediately diapered and dressed him.

"I'm sorry, Mrs. Thompson, it's been one of those nights," I apologized. "Little David has all the symptoms of Rotavirus, which has been going around recently. Be sure to give him plenty of fluids. We have some samples of Pedialyte here and I think that would be good for him. He should start to get better in a day or two. If he is unable to hold anything down, take him to the Pediatric Clinic at the University Hospital or bring him back here. Do you have any questions?"

I'm sure the look on my face was enough to deter any attempt at questioning my medical judgment or instructions. Miss James gave them a twelve pack of Pedialyte and some information on caring for babies with Rotavirus while I cleaned my shoes and rinsed my shirt.

I returned to work and was greeted by Miss James emerging from Exam Room One looking white as a ghost and holding her hand over her mouth. As the door closed an overpowering stench wafted through my nostrils and almost caused me to join my nurse who was now violently retching in the sink. The smell of fetid stool was filling our Clinic, threatening to send all of us out into the street.

"I'll open the side door, you get all the windows," I shouted as Miss James composed herself. The cool night breeze helped to carry away some of the foul odor while my intrepid nurse attacked it with a steady stream of F.O.E.

"Perirectal Abscess is draining in Room One," Miss James announced.

"I could have guessed, you know. Now all the mystery is gone," I replied. "It's things like this which make me glad I broke my nose in the fourth grade."

I looked at the chart outside Exam Room One. Eric Miller, twenty-nine, complaining of pain in the butt, otherwise healthy.

"OK, wish me luck. I'm going in," I informed Miss James.

"Wait," she said, putting her hands on my shoulders. She reached up and gave me a kiss on my cheek. "For luck, in case you don't return."

I smiled and then answered her kiss. "If I should fall in combat, please remember me; remember that I gave my life to the never-ending battle against pus."

I took a deep breath and opened the door.

"Good evening, Mr. Miller," I greeted my patient by extending my hand. "What's the problem you are having?"

Even though I was making a conscious effort to breathe only through my mouth, the powerful odor still managed to find its way into the olfactory centers of my brain. I summoned all my will power, commanding my dinner to stay put, as I faced Mr. Miller.

"I've got this terrible pain in my rectum for five days," he reported. "It started draining a little bit two days ago."

"Is that when this powerful smell started?" I inquired.

"I guess so, although I don't really notice it much," he stated, although I couldn't see how he could *not* notice it.

"Well, let me look at your bottom, although I'm sure you should be at the hospital. You're going to need surgery, at least an I&D."

"I&D?"

"Incision and drainage of the abscess I'm sure you have. It will make you feel better right away," I explained as I examined his perianal area and confirmed my diagnosis, all the time struggling to breathe.

The entire posterior and left side of the perianal area was red and hard, except for a black area in the middle. And, I was sure I felt some crepitance suggesting a particularly nasty infection.

"Are you diabetic, Mr. Miller?"

"Not that I've ever been told. But, I haven't been to a doctor in years."

"Did the nurse take any blood for testing?"

"No, but she didn't stay in the room very long. She sort of looked sick."

"Yes, she's not feeling all that well for some reason, maybe it was your special cologne. Anyway, I'll draw some blood for testing, but we need to get you to the hospital. Should I call an ambulance?"

"I'll drive myself," he decided.

"Good idea, you'll get there faster. I'll call the surgeon on call and have a crew standing by to take care of you. Good luck."

Miss James had recovered and we managed to get Mr. Miller off to University Hospital with minimal fuss. Steve Johnson was on call and he told me he'd have his residents standing by to tackle what I was sure was a case of Fournier's gangrene, although Mr. Miller didn't really look very sick. We did do a fingerstick glucose before he left and found it was 350.

A tough way to find out you're diabetic.

The powerful scent of infected necrotic tissue lingered in my nose as Miss James and I had a brief respite from our duties.

"Vomit, poop, piss, and pus; I'd say it's been a very fragrant shift, don't you agree, Nurse?"

Miss James was only barely recovering from the ordeal and gave a faint smile. The pungent scent of Mr. Miller still lingered in the air and my feeble attempt at consolation only made things worse.

"It's not that bad anymore. Maybe there's something else making you sick?" I queried.

"I'll be OK. I think I'll lie down for a few minutes. At least until another patient shows up."

"Fine, I'll man the front."

I sat at the reception desk studying the latest treatments for stage four lung cancer when an older man walked in. He looked familiar; perhaps he had been a patient in the past.

I glanced up from my journal as he signed in: M. Adams, headache. The name struck a chord in my brain, Maurice Adams as in Dr. Maurice Adams, Cardiothoracic surgeon who had retired only a few years ago. His name still struck terror in the hearts and minds of medical students and residents. He had been famous for grilling underlings rotating through his service on the finer points of anatomy and physiology.

"Just a few minutes, Dr. Adams and," I hesitated a bit, "these forms need to be filled out."

"Of course, young man," he answered as he took the clipboard and sat down in the lobby.

From my vantage point behind the reception desk something about him didn't look right.

Of course something's not right, that's why he came to the Clinic.

He looked gaunt and old, not the vigorous surgeon I remembered. Miss James came up front at that moment and took over. She looked much better, the usual color had returned to her cheeks and she even managed a smile for me.

"That's Dr. Adams. I know him from University Hospital, he was their number one heart surgeon until he retired a couple of years ago. There was some flack about him when he left, but I don't know any details."

"Well, he certainly smells better than all the other patients we've had today," she observed her nose capturing the fragrance I had missed, a flowery smell which was very appealing.

"I'm not sure what it is, but it is very pleasant and soothing, like being at home" she said.

I must have looked confused.

"Spring floral. You should know it; it's almost the same scent as those air fresheners I keep in the bathroom."

I nodded in agreement, embarrassed because I had never noticed any air fresheners.

I took a short break while Miss James ushered the eminent Dr.

Adams into Exam Room One. I glanced at his paperwork:

"Maurice Adams MD, FACS, seventy two, no allergies, no meds, no previous surgery, smokes occasional cigar, retired."

I knocked on the door, waited a few seconds, then went in.

"Good evening, Dr. Adams. I'm Dr. Barnes. You probably don't remember me, but I rotated through your service five years ago. What can I do for you?"

He eyed me up and down before answering, "Oh, yes, Dr. Barnes. I see you managed to graduate medical school, even though you once cut out one of my knots and I had to start over."

"You remember, Sir?" I'm sure I was turning red at the mention of my past misdeed. "I'm sorry about that, Sir. I was just a third-year student. But, what about you? What's the problem you are having?"

"I see you went into Internal Medicine, good choice, you'll cause less mayhem."

I was beginning to grow a little impatient. "What about you, Sir? It says you're having headaches."

"Oh, yeah," and he pressed his hands against each side of his head. "They'd almost stopped until you reminded me. I couldn't sleep, my head was pounding, like someone had hammered a seven-inch spike into each ear. I took Acetaminophen, Ibuprofen, Tramadol, oxycodone, and nothing helped. I was on my way to the hospital when I saw your sign, so I thought I'd stop here instead. Thought it might be quicker."

"Well, you are right about that, Sir. And, I have to say that after an endless stream of patients reeking of poop and vomit, your cologne is a breath of fresh air. Now, besides the headaches, any other medical problems?"

"That's why I liked cardiac surgery. Just blood, no encounters with the greasy shit pipe or mucus. Just nice, clean blood."

"Your health, Sir," I tried to direct him back to his problem.

"Nothing, no meds, no allergies, only rotator cuff surgery to fix an old golf injury."

"OK, let me take a look at you."

He winced and drew back as I moved closer to examine him. He closed his eyes and wrinkled his nose and then he took out a small vial, unscrewed the lid, and took a long sniff in each nostril. I recognized the scent as identical to the one we had noticed in the lobby.

I took out my flashlight to check his eyes. He kept them tightly closed.

"Does the light hurt your eyes?" I asked.

"A little," he replied.

"OK, I'll just look at them without the light."

I put the flashlight away and he opened his eyes. The first thing I noticed was that his pupils were unequal. The right reacted briskly as I moved my hand away from it, while the left was larger and only barely moved. As I looked more closely there was slight asymmetry of the face with the right drooping.

"How long have you been having headaches?"

"Off and on for years."

"Have they gotten worse recently?"

"I'm not sure. I know it was bad today and nothing helped. That's why I'm here. Can't you just give me a shot so I can get some relief? Then I promise I won't trouble you again."

"Just trying to be thorough, Sir, like you taught me."

I smiled at him, but he just stared straight ahead, as if I wasn't even there, like his mind was off in another world.

"I think you should have an MRI, Dr. Adams, but, for now, I'll get you a shot of Morphine..."

"No," he interrupted. "Demerol, that works better for me. Usually 75 IV does the trick."

"OK, OK, but you really need to see a Neurologist. I'll call Dr. Joint and I'm sure he'll see you tomorrow, even if it is Sunday."

"Thank you, young man. Now... Demerol."

It was more command than request and his insistent attitude made me wonder just a little about the circumstances of his "retirement."

"The nurse will be back shortly," I responded, but as I said this I saw that he was back to staring blankly into space.

I found Miss James looking like her normal cheerful self and asked her to give Dr. Adams the shot of Demerol and then went to the break room for a moment. As I rummaged around in the fridge looking for something cold to drink, I heard a loud crash. I ran to the front and heard more noises coming from the exam room. I threw the door open and found Miss James being held by Dr. Adams, a scalpel at her throat.

"Stop right there, Dr. Barnes, or I'll finish what I've started."

"Just don't do anything foolish, Dr. Adams. We'll do what you want. Just let her go."

"Oh, I will, I will let her go, once I've put an end to her misery."

I took a step towards them, but he tightened his grip on her and held the blade against her neck. At the same time I saw him wince and close his eyes for a moment. Before I could respond, however, he saw me and I took a step back. He wrinkled his nose and then he put the little vial to his nose and inhaled deeply. The floral scent reached my nose and filled the room.

"What is it, Doctor? What is going on? You don't know, do you, but I do. It's the tumor, the one in your head pushing on your brain, filling it with ugly, violent thoughts, telling you to use your surgical skills for evil. You know I'm telling you the truth. You're a doctor, you're a surgeon, you don't kill people, you save them."

"Kill people? I've never killed anyone. I perform surgery on them, make them better. Unfortunately, sometimes the patient doesn't make it." He winced again and took a sniff from the little vial.

"It's unbearable," he explained, "the smell, like feces and rotting garbage, night and day filling my head, sometimes all I can do is clench my fist and close my eyes until the worst passes. Lavender helps, it reminds me of my wife."

"Dr. Adams," I implored. "You can't do this. You're a doctor."

"I was a doctor. Now I'm famous, now I'm the Lavender Killer."

He started to cut Miss James neck, a careful, deep, even stroke right over the anterior border of the sternocleidomastoid muscle. Blood began to pour out as my nurse screamed.

"She's pregnant, you know; you'll be killing her unborn child. Could you possibly live with that?" I screamed and he stopped. Blood continued to squirt out of the wound as he dropped the scalpel. I ran to Miss James, knocking the distraught Dr. Adams aside. I grabbed a box of gauze sponges and ripped it open and applied pressure to the open wound. Luckily, this seemed to staunch the bleeding.

"Quick thinking, Dr. Barnes. It looks like you messed up another outfit," Miss James whispered, looking at my blood-stained clothes.

The bleeding had stopped and I taped the gauze dressing in place as I called 911 to report the capture of the Lavender serial killer and to call for an ambulance.

Dr. Adams was crying uncontrollably as the police cuffed him and led him away. It turned out that he had a massive tumor which was pressing on the olfactory center of his brain. He died two weeks later.

Miss James had not suffered injury to any vital structures. She recovered uneventfully and was back at work in a few weeks.

"It was quick thinking to say that I was pregnant," she commented after she was home.

"Well... I remembered that Dr. Adams always talked about how he loved children, he was always very vocal about this during his operations. I figured that the conflict created by the thought of him killing an unborn child would at least get him to stop and perhaps give me the chance to intervene. I think it worked pretty well. I mean, you are still here."

"And still pregnant."

Night Clinic Delivery

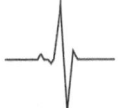

"WHAT SHOULD WE DO ABOUT IT?" I ASKED FOR THE THOU-sandth time. "I'm not even done with my training. Having a baby was definitely not in my plans. A nice cushy Dermatology fellow-ship was more what I had in mind."

"Well, you should think about such things next time you take off your pants," Miss James responded. "I did go to nursing school and it definitely takes two parties to make one baby."

"So what are you going to do?" I asked again, only leaving the we out this time.

"Well," she said with ice in her voice, "in about two hundred and thirty five days *we*, God willing, will be parents to a beautiful baby boy or girl."

She turned and walked up to the front of the Clinic to respond to the bell we both had just heard.

Me, a father? I'm barely a doctor. Well... it could be worse. I'm sure I can figure out a way to be a father with the lovely Miss James and I still be a Dermatologist. I thought I was being clever, telling that murderous Dr. Adams that Miss James was pregnant, but I guess I was more clairvoyant than clever.

"Look at this," Miss James remarked as she placed a package on the table. "It was on the reception desk, no delivery man, no mail or UPS truck, just this package. It isn't even addressed to anyone. Just this."

She tilted the package forward and showed me the white label on the top:

A.T.

To

A.P.

"Very strange, strange indeed," I observed. The package was about two feet by three feet by two feet, covered in brown wrapping paper and tied with string. It was pretty light; I almost thought it was an empty box.

"Should we open it?" my companion asked.

"I'm not sure… but there's the bell again. I guess we'll have to deal with this later. Time to go to work."

We put the package on the floor behind the table in the break room, not completely hidden, but also not in plain sight. Miss James began all the administrative paper work on our new patient while I took a few moments to look at the offers I'd recently received for Dermatology fellowships.

Southern California looks good, sun and sand… maybe Arizona, no rain, no cold weather…

"Mr. Phelps is waiting in Exam Room One, Dr. Schlemiel," Miss James announced, still with a frosty edge to her words.

I hope this doesn't go on all night.

I picked up the chart and read about Anthony Phelps. Fifty one, no allergies, no meds, chief complaint: fever and rash.

Right up my alley.

I knocked and went in and greeted Mr. Phelps with my usual bedside banter. "Good evening, Mr. Phelps, what is the problem you are having today?"

"Hello, Dr. Barnes. Tony Phelps," he rose from his chair and shook my hand. His grip was tight, a little too tight as if he was trying to establish some sort of hierarchy. "I've had a fever for several days, nothing much, 99.8, a hundred, and I've also developed a rash on my buttocks. It is quite uncomfortable."

"Just on your backside?"

"Yes."

"Did it start as a small area and spread or did it start by covering the whole area?"

"The whole area."

"Come in contact with anything unusual? Been traveling? Any allergies?"

"No, no, and no," he replied, but he looked around as he answered my questions, as if someone else was listening. Then he added, "I'm usually very healthy."

"Well, I guess I should check out the culprit. Here's a gown. Take everything off from the waist down. I'll be back in a minute."

"Before you go, Dr. Barnes, I was wondering, were any strange packages delivered here recently. I was told I might find what I'm looking for here."

"We get things delivered here all the time. Medical supplies, test results, free samples from pharmaceutical companies. What does this package look like?"

"It would be about yay big," he held his hands about twelve inches apart, "and feel like there was a jar or bottle inside."

"No, I can't say we've received any such package, at least not that I know of. Now, your gown?"

"The package may have been bigger. I was told it would be here."

"I'll tell you what," I finally said, "you put this gown on so I can finish checking you out and I will check with my nurse about your missing package, OK?"

He murmured an affirmation and I left him alone. I found Miss James checking in another patient and gestured for her to join me. She handed a very large man a clipboard to fill out and then we went to the back to look at the package. It looked smaller to me and felt a little heavier.

"Maybe this is what Mr. Phelps is looking for," Miss James concluded.

"I don't know. I get the feeling we've been drawn into some sort of international espionage. Maybe it's a 'Mission Impossible,' after all, he is Mr. Phelps. I don't think we should give him the package without some sort of proof that it's his, even if his initials are A.P."

I went back to check on my patient. He was laying face down on the table, properly attired in his gown. I pulled up the gown to see a cacophony of skin disorders all come together on his buttocks. There were patches of obvious bacterial infections, others which looked like chemical burns, reactive dermatitis, weeping sores, and petechial rashes, all limited to his derriere.

"Your buttocks are quite unusual, that is, the skin disorder you have is unusual. Are you sure you haven't come in contact with anything toxic or out of the ordinary? Because, it looks like you've been attacked by a mixture of *Strep,* acid, fire ants, and I don't know what else."

Mr. Phelps closed his eyes, pulled his gown over his butt, and turned towards me. He looked a bit sheepish.

"It's hard to explain, Dr. Barnes. In my line of work there is the potential to come in contact with a variety of toxins and poisons, dangerous chemical and biological agents. One way to deal with this is to intentionally expose oneself to these noxious materials to build up a sort of immunity or at least a tolerance. I think I tried to do too much at one time."

"What are you some kind of secret agent or a garbage collector? Well, I suppose it doesn't matter, there isn't much difference between the two anyway. I'll give you a prescription for some antibiotics and some cream to put on your backside. Try it for three or four days. If you're better, fine, but if you're not improving, come back." I gave him a prescription for Cipro and another for some antifungal, antibacterial steroid cream.

"Check out with Miss James at the front, and if there's no improvement, come back here or see your own doctor."

"Thank you, Dr. Barnes. You've been very helpful," Mr. Phelps replied as I escorted him to the front.

I left him to look at the chart of my next patient, the very large man I'd seen in the waiting room. K. Gutman, no age listed, no medical problems, no allergies, chief complaint shortness of breath, blood pressure 180/95. I was about to go when I felt the pocket of my white coat and realized I didn't have my stethoscope.

Must have left it in the break room.

I heard some rustling and furniture moving as I approached the break room entrance. I stopped and peeked inside and saw a man in a beige raincoat bending over behind the table. When he stood up I saw that it was Mr. Phelps, now holding our mysterious package.

"I've been searching for this for years. Never would have thought it'd turn up in some rinky dink medical clinic in the middle of the city," he commented as he put the package under his arm.

"Do you think it's safe for you to just walk out of here carrying that bundle? Don't you think they've been following you?" I answered.

Phelps looked around, up and down, towards the window, inside his coat, and then he put the package back behind the table.

"You're right; they're probably watching me right now; probably don't believe that I would come to this Clinic with a real medical condition."

He stroked his chin as he thought. "I'll tell you what. You keep it here, keep it safe. I'll give them the slip and then come back for it."

He didn't wait for me to answer. He put on a pair of dark glasses and snuck out the back of the Clinic. I shrugged my shoulders, found my stethoscope, and went back to see Mr. Gutman.

Gutman, that name sounds familiar.

"Good evening, Mr. Gutman, my name is Dr. Barnes. What's the problem that brings you into our wonderful little Clinic?" I began.

"Nice to see you, Doctor. I will dispense with the usual pleasantries and get straight to the point," he replied.

Great. When someone says they'll get straight to the point, they usually do everything but get straight to the point.

Gutman was big, rotund, with beads of sweat dotting his forehead. He was dressed in a finely tailored gray suit and I detected a slight accent in his voice.

"I've been having trouble catching my breath, Dr. Barnes. I first noticed it on the train from Istanbul to Prague. Since then I've noticed that I have to stop and rest on a regular basis."

"Have you seen a doctor before?"

"No, I haven't have had the time. I frequently have to leave one venue for another on very short notice and doctors have not fit into my busy calendar. Fortunately, my travels have brought me to your Clinic and so I thought I would 'kill two birds with one stone' as you Americans so quaintly articulate."

"Well, it's good that you stopped here. Your blood pressure is very high and I can see that you are dangerously overweight."

"Yes, yes, one of the consequences of living one's life from hotel to train to cruise ship and back to hotels. One never gets the proper opportunity to exercise or to eat healthily."

"I think you've done a bit too much eating, healthily or unhealthily."

"Harrumph," was all he could say so I continued.

"Your blood pressure is dangerously elevated, you have bilateral carotid artery bruits which suggests to me that you are heading for a serious stroke. You have wheezing in both lungs and your legs look like tree trunks. In short, you are a walking time bomb. I recommend you start on a medically supervised diet and medication for your blood pressure. We need to get the results of your blood work, also. I'm betting your sugar will be high which means you're probably diabetic. We can manage your health problems here at the Clinic or you can follow up with your own doctor. But, I would not ignore these medical conditions, that is, if you want to live beyond the next six months or so."

"My dear, Dr. Barnes," he responded, "I am grateful for your concern, but these 'medical problems' are mere trifles in the grand scheme of this world. I have been in pursuit of a truly remarkable and valuable treasure and I have followed it to your Clinic. I believe a package was delivered here earlier?"

I didn't answer, but I think he could tell from the look on my face that he was correct.

"This package, Sir, is one that I have been following for many years. I thought I had finally secured it in Oslo three years ago, but, at the last moment it eluded my grasp, only to resurface in Cairo. My contact there met with an unfortunate accident before he could make delivery. I've since chased this prize through every corner of the continent and now it has turned up in your medical clinic. As one can easily surmise, Sir, I have spent a considerable sum of money chasing this prize. And, if you were to be so kind as to deliver it to me, I would pay you handsomely for your brief troubles."

I looked at him and saw the combination of greed and desperation in his loose jowls and pig-like eyes.

"What, if I may be so bold as to ask, is in this little package?"

"A magnificent bird, fourteen inches tall, made of solid gold and bejeweled with perfect diamonds, emeralds, rubies, and sapphires. It was a gift to the ruler of the Ottoman Turks in 1647, but was lost in 1800. It reappeared briefly in London in the 1820's and also was held by a private collector in Paris some years later. It was taken by the Nazi's during the occupation and was thought lost forever, a victim of the war. It was only after the fall of the Soviet Union that it resurfaced, first in Moscow, then Budapest."

"This bird manages to make it all over Europe," I commented. Gutman only raised his eyebrows slightly at my remark.

"I have it on very reliable information that the package which was delivered, quite mistakenly to your Clinic, is the priceless falcon. And now, Dr. Barnes, I will take that package. If you would be so kind as to bring it here."

I was staring at a pistol.

Why do I feel like Humphrey Bogart? Give him his package; it's prob-

ably a fake anyway.

"OK, OK, I'll get it for you. It's been nothing but trouble since it arrived anyway. Don't forget, however, that you need to look after yourself. Remember, if you don't have your health, you don't have anything."

I went to the break room and found the package behind the table where I'd left it. As I started to bring it to Gutman, Miss James stopped me.

"Where are you taking our mysterious box?" she wondered.

"Mr. Gutman says it belongs to him and he has a nine millimeter handgun that makes it difficult for me to argue."

"Oh," was all she said. "Probably for the best anyway. It has been nothing but trouble."

I picked the box up and noticed that it was much heavier than I remembered.

Solid gold bird would be pretty heavy.

I started to hand the box to Gutman who was sitting on the exam table. He had more sweat on his forehead and his head was bent down and he was struggling to breathe. The pistol was hanging on two fingers and crashed to the floor followed shortly by Mr. Gutman.

"Mr. Gutman… Mr. Gutman, can you hear me?" I asked. He was still breathing and his eyes were looking around the room as if he was trying to remember where he was.

"The bird," he whispered, "do you have it? May I see it?"

"I have the package here. I'll put it in your arms," I answered. I gently lay the package across his chest and folded his arms around it. He held it tightly to his chest and a smile graced his face.

"At last, at last, after years and years of …" his voice trailed off.

Miss James was already there with the crash cart as Kasper Gutman breathed his last breath. We performed CPR and the ambulance arrived, all to no avail. With considerable effort they managed to get him onto a stretcher. I even thought we had brought him back, but then he went back into V. Fib and then asystole.

I put the cursed package back in the break room and then filled out all the paperwork which is required if someone dies at the Clinic. The Coroner's assistant arrived and carted Gutman away and that was that.

"Anyone else waiting Miss Ja...?" I started to ask but was interrupted by a person dressed in black medieval armor, holding a long, shiny, sharp sword gracefully pointed at my heart.

"I will take the Grail," the muffled voice commanded.

"Grail?" I asked, my voice filled with confusion.

"The Holy Grail. I saw it delivered here today. I've been on a quest to retrieve it for years and years. Now, young sir, you shall deliver it to me or suffer the consequences. Perhaps," he mused, "I shall run you through just for the sport of it and then take my prize anyway.

They don't pay me enough for this.

"I'm sure I don't know what you are talking about. This is a Medical Clinic. We take care of sick people here. We don't have any grails."

He pushed his sword against my chest, then raised it above his head as he prepared to run me through. As his arm moved forward and I closed my eyes, I heard a loud "CLANG" as metal struck metal.

A second knight, this one clad in silver armor, had appeared.

"Forsooth and avast, ye wicked Black Knight. You shall never possess the Holy Grail as long as I can draw a breath," the Silver Knight shouted.

Avast? Don't pirates say that?

My attention returned to the ensuing battle.

"Sir Lancelot, you are more relentless than I imagined. But the Holy Grail shall be mine."

Swords clanged together as the two knights battled from one end of the clinic waiting room to the other. Chairs were slashed, potted plants upended and magazines strewn about.

A very large woman came in as the sword fight raged. She walked past the two knights, ignoring the combat, to the reception desk.

"Ya'll open?" she asked in a very demanding voice. "Cuz my back is killin' me and I can't get no sleep."

I stared at her and then at the two combatants and then back at her.

She saw the confused look on my face, but went right on talking.

"Listen up, Dr....Barnes," she stared at my ID badge, "when I'm talkin' to you, you pays me propa attention. That fightin' goes on all the time in this neighborhood, but I'sa hurtin' and you got's to do somethin'."

I turned my attention to her. "Certainly, Ms...."

"Angelina, just like Angelina Jolie. Angelina Babbett. Like I was sayin', my back is sore like someone's stickin' a knife."

"OK, Ms. Jolie, I mean Babbett. Fill out these forms and we'll get you right back."

She took the clipboard and sat down while Lancelot and the Black Knight fought on. The clanging of metal mixed with Ms. Babbett's murmuring as she answered the pages of questions. Every time a chair was knocked over or there was an especially loud crash she looked up and gave the knights an especially dirty look. Finally, she couldn't stand it anymore. She jumped up from her seat and rapped the Black Knight on his helmet with the clipboard. The fighting stopped abruptly as both surprised Knights stared at her.

"You two good fo' nuthin's get yo asses out o' my way. My back is killing me and I canna get this here paper filled out with all that there racket. You got fightin' to do, you does it outside and leave this here clinic fo' the sick folks."

I approached Lancelot.

"I'll keep it safe for you, right here. You go battle the Black Knight and defeat him and then you can come back for the Grail."

"Excellent plan, young doctor. But, be sure to keep it safe or it shall be you I will pursue."

"I promise I will treat the package with all the respect and care it deserves." And I opened the door and ushered him out. The Black Knight had already made his escape and when Lancelot saw his adversary riding away he made a hasty exit and mounted his armored horse.

"Au revoir, good doctor," he shouted as he rode away.

I have to admit it was quite a sight, two men in full armor, each astride an equally armored horse, racing down the street with swords raised, illuminated by the pale light of the street lamps. I turned away, shaking my head.

This box... this mysterious box. I don't think I want to know what's really inside. It's going to get us killed.

"Miss Babbett is waiting in Room One. I suspect a shot of Dilaudid will send her on her way," Miss James reported from the doorway.

I looked again towards Lancelot and the Black Knight as they faded into the night and then turned and headed back into the Clinic.

"Do you think we should open it?" Miss James asked.

"Perhaps," was all I could say. I thought for a few more moments. "I think I know what we would find inside. We would be disappointed."

"Do you think it's empty?" she wondered out loud.

"I think it's full and empty and everything in between."

"Please, don't speak in riddles," she replied.

"I have no choice because that little package is just that... a riddle. 'A.T. to A. P.' is a riddle. Now, I'm going to see poor Miss Babbett and maybe you can solve the riddle while you're waiting."

Before I could escape to the Exam Room, a quartet waltzed through the door; an unusual group, even for the Clinic.

"If you please, Sir, I believe there is a package here that would be of great benefit to us," said the little girl.

Why am I not surprised.

Standing at the reception desk were Dorothy, the Scarecrow, the Tin Man, and the Cowardly Lion.

The Scarecrow explained, "We've been following that box all the way from Oz. It's the only thing that will give me a brain or the Tin Man his heart…"

"Or me my courage," the Lion chimed in.

"And it will help Dorothy find her way home," the Tin Man added.

"Now wait a minute, wait a minute," I replied. "I do believe that the Wizard was supposed to have granted all your requests."

"The Wizard? You mean the Charlatan, the humbug," Scarecrow answered. "Do you really believe that a fake diploma from some fake 'university' qualifies as a brain? I was laughed right out of the cornfield when I showed it to one of the crows. That crow said he was smarter than me and stole all of my corn just to prove it."

"And that heart?" the Tin Man added, followed by a sigh. "I was so careful with it, kept it around my neck right over my chest. Five days after he gave it to me, it started running backwards and then it went 'fhht' followed by complete cardiac arrest, if you get my meaning. If I was dependent on it to pump blood I'd be face down in the gutter. Hmmph, how could I be duped to think a two-dollar drug store clock is as good as a Jarvik seven."

"That medal was nice," The Lion said in a soft, almost embarrassed voice, "although it hurt when he pinned it on."

"Yes, yes, very nice and what did it get you? The first time you tried to stand up to another beast, they laughed and that was just a squirrel. What did you do?" Dorothy asked.

"Please, don't tell, don't…"

"He runs away and hides in the bushes; some courage. And, I guess it's clear that I am not in Kansas, Dr….Barnes."

"Yes, this is definitely not Kansas. Just what makes you think that this box you're looking for has all these things which you desire?"

"It must, we were promised. I sold my ruby slippers to get what's in that box. The man promised."

"Someone from around here?" I surmised.

"Yes, he had a black coat and an ID that said he was from the government and would help us," she answered meekly.

They can have it, the stupid box. It's been only trouble.

"Well the box is here and you are welcome to it. Just wait here and I'll fetch it for you."

I went to the back to retrieve the troublesome parcel. I looked behind the table, but there was no box. I looked under and around and over every nook and cranny: no box. I went to find Miss James, but she had no idea where the box disappeared to.

Miss Babbett was standing in the doorway to the Exam Room and saw us searching high and low.

"Looking for something?" she inquired.

"There was a package back here, wrapped in brown paper about so big," Miss James explained.

"You mean that the stinky box that was in that room back there? I throwed it away. I couldna' stand the stench, almos' made me to vomick. It's in the garbage dumpster. Now what about my back?"

"I'll be right back and take care of you," I said as I ran towards the back of the Clinic.

It was getting late, almost 5:30 and this was garbage day. I heard the roar of a truck in the alley and ran outside just in time to see the garbage truck driving away. I peered over the edge of the dumpster and saw only a few dirty rags which had clung to the bottom. I went back to inform Dorothy and her companions.

"I'm terribly sorry, Miss Gale, but the package you are seeking is gone. It was inadvertently thrown away and now it's on that garbage truck which you can see down the street. I pointed to the truck and, before I could say another word, the four raced away after it. I went inside to take care of Ms. Barrett just as a big RV pulled up. There was a colorful logo painted on its side:

JASON AND THE ARGONAUTS

I've heard of them, some sort of rock group.

A solidly built young man emerged from the door on the RV's side and came inside.

"I'm Jason, lead singer for the Argonauts. I was told I might find something here, something I've been searching for…"

I stopped and stared into his eyes. He was tall with blonde hair and a dark complexion.

"If you're looking for the Golden Fleece you are about five minutes too late. If you hurry you can probably catch it. It's in that garbage truck you just passed. Just look for a truck being chased by a little girl, a scarecrow, tin man, and lion."

"Thank you, Doctor." And he turned and walked out.

I went back to the Exam Room to tend to my patient.

"That ther' box sho did stink. Almos' made me fogit about thes here back pain. But, now it's a throbbin agin. Musta bin some sort of dead possum or rottin' trash in thet package."

"How long have you been having back pain, Ms. Barrett?" I asked, trying to focus on her problems.

"Wha was in thet ther' box anyways? Do you knows?" she wondered.

I stopped and thought for a moment, staring off into the distance.

"Dreams, Ms. Barrett, lost and unfulfilled dreams," I replied in a soft voice.

She looked at me as if I had lost my mind.

"But, for you, I think a shot of Dilaudid will work just fine and then you can follow up at the Back Clinic over at County Hospital."

"Demerol woks better," she interjected.

"OK, Demerol."

"Seventy five IV."

"OK, OK."

Miss James gave her the medication and we sent her on her

way.

Afterwards it was just the two of us alone in the Clinic.

"What are you thinking?" although I didn't really need to ask.

"That box; so much hope wrapped up in a plain brown wrapper. Do you think any of them will ever find what they are looking for?"

"I suppose they'll all find something and, in the end, they will probably be disappointed. It's the anticipation of something better which keeps us going. How often are we let down in the end? But, back to 'A.T. to A.P.' What is the answer?"

"You keep thinking about it, Dr. Barnes, that's what you're best at," Miss James commented, but then she patted her belly. "Well, I have to admit, you are good at a few other things, too."

NIGHT CLINIC MUSE

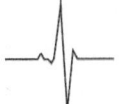

Swing Low, sweet Chariot
Coming for to carry me home
Swing Low Sweet Chariot
Coming for to carry me home

I WALKED INTO THE CLINIC AND WAS GREETED BY THESE gospel strains delivered by my lovely nurse.

"I never knew you had such a sweet voice, charming nurse," I complimented her. "Is it only gospel or do you do rock and roll, too?"

"Jazz, blues, or gospel, fine doctor, but I usually only sing when no one's around. Performing was never my strong suit. My muse only visits when I'm alone."

"Too bad, really. You really have an amazing voice. All we have to do is get you discovered and I wouldn't have to slave away at the Hospital or here at the Clinic."

"Don't get your hopes up, Dr. Barnes. I'm a nurse first and foremost. Although, maybe, if you're lucky, I'll sing for you in the shower."

"I'm not sure all three of us can fit in the shower together."

"Three?"

"Me, you, and your belly."

"I guess if we stand real close we could swing it," she concluded after a bit of thought. "But, cleanliness comes later. Right now Albee D'Amico is in Room One. Something about loss of balance or equilibrium."

"Just what I need to start the night. An unbalanced individual. OK, Mr. D'Amico, ready or not, I'm comin' in."

I knocked and entered Room One, "Good evening, Mr. D'Amico, I'm Dr. Barnes. What is the problem you are having?"

I heard a low hum as I walked in and found my patient sitting cross-legged on the table, arms at his side, eyes closed, and a steady humming coming from his closed mouth.

"Excuse me, Mr. D'Amico," I said softly, nudging him on the shoulder, "are you OK? What can I do for you?"

He opened one eye, looked at me, then closed his eye and went back to his humming.

"Fine," I announced. "If you're not sick, you don't need to be here. You can do your meditation or Karma or whatever you call it somewhere else." And I started to leave.

Before I could go too far, his arm shot out and he grabbed my wrist, all the while continuing his incessant, annoying chant.

I tried to shake my arm loose, but he had a very powerful grip.

"My Muse," he whispered. "I've lost her and I think she's here. I'm trying to get her back. I need to get her back."

He relaxed his hold on my wrist and I pulled away, shaking my hand to restore the feeling.

"Mr. D'Amico, I am truly sorry that you have lost your Muse, but I do not see how I can help you. This is a medical clinic, not an artist's retreat," I stated emphatically.

"But," he retorted with a little more force in his voice, my Muse has left me because of a medical problem, I'm sure of it. Therefore, if you give me a complete going over, I am sure you will discover the malady which has left me with this forlorn feeling of abandonment. Then, my confidence restored, I shall be able to return to my work."

"And what, may I ask, is your work?"

"I write songs, that is, I write song lyrics. I was in the process of writing the lyrics for a new jazz album when she left. Since then I've barely been able to write my name."

"OK, Mr. D'Amico, I'll give you a check up. But tell me, when did your Muse desert you?"

"Tuesday, a week ago, at 3:11 a.m. She just packed up and left. I searched all over my apartment and in the alley and even by the lake in the park, which is where she hides sometimes, but nothing. Finally, I went to see Madam Tahini."

"Madam Tahini?"

"You know, Madam Tahini, over at Tahini's Fortune Telling and Auto Repair. She told me to come here. She told me she saw my Muse right in front of this Clinic and then Madam saw the impish sprite enter the Clinic through an upstairs window. Madam told me that if I came here to have a medical check up, then that old Muse would take pity on me and come back."

I've heard sillier stories, that's for sure, but this one is still a doozy.

"OK, OK, so I'll check you out. Let's start at the beginning. What is it that brought you in here today. No, wait, let me start from different angle. Is anything hurting you or bothering you, Mr. D'Amico?"

"My head, my head feels like it's been stuffed with three weeks of dirty laundry. And my legs, they get muscle spasms every night and, let's see, my stomach. I get cramps and diarrhea almost every day."

"That's quite a lot of symptoms. How long has all this been going on?"

"Let's see. Leg cramps, eight years. Stomach pain and diarrhea, three, no four years. Headache, two days. But my chanting and meditating almost made my head feel normal, at least until you interrupted me and now it hurts again, particularly right here."

He pointed to his frontal sinus area.

"Take any medicine?"

"I don't like to poison my body with manmade, artificial concoctions. I prefer my meditation."

"How does that work for you?"

"Quite well, most of the time, unless I'm interrupted."

"Sorry about that, but you did come to the Clinic and it is my job to try to treat you."

"If you want to help me feel better, you'll start searching this building for my Muse. She's here somewhere, I can feel it."

"OK, let me finish my exam and then I'll have a look around."

So, I checked him from top to bottom and found nothing unusual. Miss James drew basic labs and we left him to await the results while I went on to the next patient.

"S. Dixon, 67, abscess left arm," I murmured as I read over the chart.

Probably a drug addict.

"Good evening, Mr. Dixon, I'm Dr. Barnes. What is the problem that brings you in here tonight?" I asked.

"Santana," he replied, standing up to shake my hand, "but, please, call me 'Wild.' It's short for 'Wild Fingers.' That's what they used to call me when I was playing."

I looked at him, eyeing him up and down. He was tall, about six four, gaunt, wearing dark glasses, blue jeans, a black t-shirt, and a black cap. There was a dirty rag taped to his left forearm.

"Wild Fingers Dixon? The guitar player?" I wondered out loud.

"You've heard of me?"

"You, Sir, are a great jazz guitarist. But, I haven't seen anything of yours for, I don't know, ten years?"

"That would be about right. My Muse left me, replaced by heroin and now, here I am, at the Free Clinic, getting treated for the consequences of my sordid life."

"I heard you play back in 1990 at the Arena. You were great; made me want to be a guitar player. Only problem I had was lack of talent. So, I ended up in medical school instead. I still try to pick at it on occasion."

"Well, I haven't picked up my guitar in years. All I can play now is a needle. Look at this arm.

He held up his arm and ripped of the makeshift bandage. There were brownish tracks up and down and an angry, red area oozing pus just below his shoulder.

"I don't think I could even hold a guitar with this arm, it hurts so bad. Therefore, I would appreciate it if you could lance this nasty abscess and just forget about ancient history."

"Well, there is no question that abscess needs to be cleaned up and you'll need to be on some antibiotics, but I think you could get back to playing once the infection is better."

As I was giving him my medical opinion, I heard some thumping and what almost sounded like footsteps coming from the ceiling above us.

Probably rats or squirrels.

But, the noise gave me an idea.

"Hear that?" I asked.

Wild nodded his head.

"That, Mr. Wild Fingers Dixon, is a Muse, your Muse as a matter of fact. The local soothsayer, Madame Tahini, assured me just this evening that the wayward Muse has taken up residence in this very Clinic. I think he or she knew you'd be here tonight and came here to be reunited."

"You're crazy," was his answer, "and I'm not sure I want a deranged psycho of a doctor touching my arm."

"Well, that *is* up to you, but, what if I'm right, think of the possibilities. How about you let me drain your abscess while you consider that you may have an opportunity to get your life, your true, intended life back. I don't think you'll have anything to lose."

"Fix my arm and then we'll talk."

"Deal."

I went to work, swabbing his arm with antiseptic solution and then did my best to numb the area. Finally, I sliced through the angry skin with a #11 scalpel. Grayish green pus under pressure shot out and spattered over my face (luckily I was wearing a mask) and then oozed out onto the sterile drape which covered his arm. I gathered some of the nasty fluid into a sterile container to be sent to the lab and then did my best to probe the abscess, looking for pockets of undrained pus.

To his credit, Wild Fingers sat still while I poked around, even though I knew it had to hurt even with the local anesthesia.

I finished as quickly as I could, like the surgeons of old, and packed and dressed the big open wound I had created.

"Wait here for a few minutes," I instructed. "I need to come back and check the dressing to be sure there isn't any bleeding. Prop it up on this pillow for now and keep it elevated as much as possible over the next few days. I'll be back in about five minutes."

I went out and found Miss James. Before I could say a word, she asked me if I'd heard noises coming from the ceiling.

"As a matter of fact, I did, so did Wild Fingers," I replied.

"Wild Fingers?" she asked.

"The patient in Room Two, Mr. Dixon. He used to be a well known jazz guitarist, before heroin wiped away his confidence. I told him it was his Muse making the noise. After all, Madame Tahini did tell our other patient that a Muse had taken up residence in our humble Clinic."

"Perhaps you should go investigate. Maybe you can sneak up on it and catch it in a bag or something. Then it will have to grant you three wishes."

"I believe that is a genie or a leprechaun. Muses inspire us to create great art or music or poetry."

"Well, whatever is up there, it has not done a very good job keeping its presence a secret. Maybe it wants to be found. Think about it; what good is a Muse if it has no one to inspire."

I went to the back of the Clinic and pulled down the retractable stairway which led to the attic. I found the flashlight we kept for emergencies and armed myself with a syringe filled with Versed and a short, heavy metal IV pole.

I ascended the staircase/ladder and entered the dusty attic over our Clinic. I searched for the light switch and found it on a wooden post, flicked it on, and nothing happened. I flicked and jiggled it back and forth without any more success.

I guess it's just me and my flashlight.

As I was fiddling with the light switch I felt a light touch on my shoulder, which made me wheel around suddenly and raise my metal weapon above my head, only to discover Miss James standing behind me.

"You shouldn't sneak up like that. I could have hurt the baby and you shouldn't be up here anyway. It's musty and dank and who knows what diseases have wafted up into these rafters over the years," I admonished.

"I thought you could use some moral support and you forgot to bring a bag. Besides, I'm not afraid of any old rat or squirrel. After all, you're armed to the teeth. I know that a syringe filled with Versed always strikes fear into my heart."

"Ha… ha," I huffed as I pointed the flashlight towards the end of the garret. "Do you hear that? That gnawing, grinding noise? I'll bet it's a big rat gnawing on some wires or something."

Miss James didn't respond so I turned and shined my light towards her, only to find the source of the noise was my companion propped up against the wall frantically scratching her leg.

"I can't help it," she whispered, "I'm pregnant and I have a terrible itch."

Let it go, don't make a fuss about it, not with a pregnant woman.

"Thump, thump, boing."

"Did you hear *that*?" she whispered in my ear. "That was not me. It came from up there." She pointed to the bare rafters.

I shined my light and saw *it*, at least for a moment. It was white, about three feet tall, and had jumped from one cross beam to another.

"Did you see it? Did you see that little thing?" I asked, hissing between clenched teeth.

"There it goes," Miss James shouted and pointed to the end of the attic.

We moved as quickly as we could towards it, but found only empty space. I shined my flashlight up and down and all around, but saw nothing. Whatever had been there was gone, vanished completely.

"Where'd it go? It was here, I know it," I exclaimed.

"Wait, there it is, on that beam," Miss James replied. "Maybe if you can scare it or surprise it, it will jump away and I can catch it in this."

She held up the red biological waste bag.

"I think it's big enough," I observed. "Shh… it's sitting over there. Quick, give me that bag."

I stared at our adversary for a minute. All I could see was a white apparition crouching on the floor, seemingly oblivious or uncaring of our presence. In the dim light I couldn't tell if it was an animal or small person or demon. I took out my trusty syringe filled with Versed and opened the bag as I crept up behind it. I stopped for a moment as the opening scene of the Ghostbusters creeping up on the ghost of the Librarian filled my head. I shook my head and continued my stealth approach.

I was standing right behind it. I quickly jabbed it in the neck with my syringe and pumped it full of Versed and then pulled the bag over its head and scooped it up. There was some brief movement until the Versed kicked in and then it went limp.

"It won't be able to breathe in that plastic bag," Miss James remarked.

"Let's get downstairs and we'll cut some holes in the bag so the little beast won't suffocate."

It wasn't heavy at all and we quickly descended the stairs back into the Clinic. I poked a few holes in the side of the bag, taking extra care not to harm our captive. I was dying of curiosity. I knew our imprisoned being was not a rat or squirrel, but I still had no idea what or who it was.

"Wait here while I go check on our patients," I told Miss James. I had almost forgotten about Wild Fingers and Mr. D'Amico.

I found them both patiently waiting. Wild Fingers' I&D site was dry and he said his pain was much improved.

Mr. D'Amico smiled as I entered his Exam Room.

"Did my lab tests tell you anything?" he asked.

"Oh, sh… I forgot," I blurted out, slapping myself on the forehead. "I'll be back in a second."

"No rush," he answered, "I've been doodling here and even came up with a few ideas."

I noticed a pile of little pieces of paper on the exam table next to him as I went to the back to check on his lab results and on Miss James and our prisoner.

I found both of them sitting at the break room table. The red bag "prison" lay empty while I saw a tiny little girl sitting on Miss James' lap, her small white arms wrapped around my nurse's neck.

"She's not feeling well, " Miss James announced. "It seems that someone filled her full of Versed and now she's got a terrible headache."

"She being…?" I inquired.

"Muse," came the reply. "It would appear that Madam Tahini was actually right. This little girl's name is Muse."

"Is she really a Muse, as in 'I will inspire the artist in you to create new and wonderful things'? Or, is it just a name?"

The little girl gave me a dirty look as she rocked back and forth in Miss James' lap.

"I don't feel artistically inspired," I continued, making a bigger ass of myself. "What I am inspired to do is find the results of Mr. D'Amico's lab so that I can send him on his way."

Both Nurse and Muse gave me a silent look that told me I was on my own, so I went into the computer and found what I was looking for.

"CBC, chem, UA, all normal, no, WBC is… shoot," I murmured.

I started back to the front to talk with Mr. D'Amico and met Miss James and Muse leaving the break room.

"We are going to see Wild Fingers. Muse told me she used to be a close friend, but she hasn't heard from him in years."

"Look at this," I interrupted and showed Miss James the CBC

result.

"Can that be correct?"

"I think it is. I'm going to talk to him now."

The bell sounded telling us there was a new patient up front, which caused Miss James to detour from the exam rooms while she did a quick evaluation of the patient in the lobby.

She called me immediately, before I could go back to see Mr. D'Amico. I found a tall, thin man with long hair and a long beard holding out his hand, which was impaled on a broken drumstick.

"I don't think I can fill out any forms with my hand like this," our new patient concluded.

"I'm inclined to agree, Mr..." I replied.

"Green, Huxley Green."

"Are you a drummer, Mr. Green?" Miss James asked.

"I am. I do a lot of studio work and play with a few bands around town. Lots of rock and country, not as much jazz as I'd like. I was practicing an hour or so ago and I had a little accident."

"I can see that. Well, it's not bleeding and your hand function seems to be intact," I noted after a quick hallway exam. "So, if you can please wait here in Room Three; Miss James, will get some information and I'll be back in a few minutes."

I left him and went back to give Mr. D'Amico some bad news.

He was still scribbling on bits of paper, now with more vigor than ever, when I entered.

"Mr. D'Amico," I said in a slightly hushed tone, "I've got the results of your blood tests."

He continued to write for a moment and then slowly looked up at me, staring into my eyes.

I continued, "Your white blood cell count is very high. Normally, a white blood cell count is less than ten thousand. If there is an infection it will go up sometimes as high as twenty five or even thirty thousand. Yours, however, is one hundred fifty thousand and all the cells are one type. What this all means is that you probably have..."

"Leukemia," he answered for me.

"You knew?" I asked.

"No, but I'm not stupid. I can read and I've seen 'Love Story.' I know what a very, very high white blood cell count means. Pity, really, because I've been nothing but inspired while I've been here."

"It must be because of Muse," I concluded.

"Muse?"

"It would seem that Madam Tahini was right, for once. We found her in the attic. A little girl…"

"…dressed in white," he finished my statement again.

"Would you stop doing that, please," I said, half joking. "How did you know?"

"I've always dreamt that my Muse was a little girl dressed in white."

"Well, she's here and I guess she's inspired you. Look at all you've accomplished."

"It's just jazz nonsense."

"You shouldn't be so modest. This is pretty good," I remarked as I deciphered some of his scribbling. "But, back to the health problem at hand."

"What type of leukemia do you think it is?" my patient wondered. "Can you tell if it's lymphocytic, myelogenous, acute, or chronic?

"For a songwriter you seem to know a lot about medicine," I observed.

"My father died of leukemia when he was fifty five. I was fifteen at the time. I made quite a study on leukemia. He had acute myelogenous leukemia. He was diagnosed on a Thursday and died on a Thursday three weeks later. At least today is Friday, otherwise this leukemia thing would definitely be a bad omen. Now, if you don't mind, I'm going to sit here, cross my legs, and meditate on all you've told me."

"That's fine. I need to tend to a drummer with a part of drumstick stuck through his hand anyway. I'll be back in few minutes and we can talk about referring you to the Leukemia section at the Cancer Hospital."

I left him alone and went back to see Huxley Green. Muse joined me as I exited the Exam Room. She looked up at me, her green eyes growing wider as she stared into my eyes. I didn't feel any sense of inspiration. I looked at the chart hanging outside the door: Huxley Green, 52, no medical problems, no allergies, accident with drumstick.

"Good evening again, Mr. Green. Can you tell me how you managed to impale your right hand on that broken drumstick?"

"I was running through a few ba-da-ba-bing and then some be-bop-a-boom and more ba-da-ba-boom when I just couldn't quite hit that phat-de-bop-bop the way I wanted. I kept tryin' though and, man, after ten whacks at it, I jumps up and I just screams, breaks the sticks in two, and chucks 'em across the room. Well, after five I calmed down a bit and gets up to clean up. Well, this here stick was sticking up in the air, I trips and wham bam I falls and here I am."

"A tragic accident I can see," I replied, "but maybe you missed everything important."

I examined his hand. Motor function looked to be normal, sensation was intact, no swelling, pink with normal capillary refill. I looked at the X-Ray Miss James had so efficiently obtained and, except for the faint shadow of the wooden drumstick, the bones all looked normal.

"I am going to do something quite bold here, Mr. Green. Just look away for a moment."

As he turned his head, I took hold of the blunt end of the drumstick and pulled. With very little effort the wooden stick slid right out and Mr. Green was cured. The holes in his hand almost closed up before my eyes as the tissue had been more spread than cut.

"I'm going to wash this out a bit, put in a couple of stitches, give you a tetanus shot and a script for antibiotics and you should be good to go. I went to work and cleaned him up and bandaged the injured hand.

As I put on the last piece of tape we both heard the same sounds. The sweet strain of guitar riffs and the bluesy voice of Miss James. I left my patient for the moment and went out to the lobby to find Miss James and Wild Fingers Dixon jamming.

Night Clinic Blues, we're livin' through
The Night Clinic Blues
The sick and the dyin' they bring us to
The Night Clinic Blues

The gangs they's a fightin over
The Night Clinic Blues
The children are ill, with fever and chill
Oh, Night Clinic Blues

And the song went on, punctuated by Wild Fingers' distinctive guitar riffs. There was an empty drum set, but not for long as Huxley Green climbed into the seat and added his potent bop-de-bop. I saw Mr. D'Amico nodding approvingly and, sitting on the reception desk was Muse, smiling.

I sat down next to D'Amico.

"We need a horn and a saxophone to really make the sound," he said.

As if on cue, the door opened and a man and a woman, Buddy and Cici, walked in, each carrying a small suitcase. Without a word, they opened their bags, the woman pulled out a trumpet, the man a saxophone, and they joined in, improvising along with Wild Fingers and Huxley as Miss James continued her throaty, bluesy song.

It don't matter if it's your heart or your head
Those Night Clinic Blues
We'll see you, we'll cure you,
Oh, Night Clinic Blues

I moved over and leaned on the desk next to Muse.

"You've done wonderful work here tonight, little Muse," I whispered in her ear.

She just turned to me and smiled.

"Can you inspire me to be a greater doctor?" I wondered.

And then she spoke, the only words I heard her say that night. "Medicine is as much an art as singing or playing the drums. But, it is not my place to inspire you; you have your own muse. Just don't be surprised if she comes to you at the most unusual moments. I need to leave here, but you will see me again. Your child will become my good friend."

A smile came to my face as I thought about "my child" for a few minutes and then as I turned to respond to her words, she jumped off the desk and ran across the lobby and into the arms of a tall, blonde, elegant woman, also dressed in white, who was standing just inside the door. This woman picked her up, gave her a kiss on the cheek, and they left.

I ran after them, but outside the street was empty.

There were no more patients that shift, so I enjoyed the rest of the concert. Buddy and Cici left before dawn. Wild Fingers and Mr. D'Amico hung around for a bit longer trying to convince Miss James to join them in the local jazz clubs.

"I don't see how I can," she answered. "I'm due to deliver in a couple of months and then I'll be a mother *and* a nurse. Perhaps Cici can take over the singing chores."

I set up a referral for Mr. D'Amico to be seen at the Leukemia Clinic and called University Hospital Rehab and made arrangements for Wild Fingers to check in later that day.

Miss James and I had a few minutes to ourselves before it was time for the next crew to arrive.

"You are very good," I remarked. "Your singing, I mean. You should be on one of those singing reality shows, like American Idol."

"I could never do that," she replied. "Singing in front of you and the others was more than I could usually do; it was all I could do to keep from throwing up. I think it was Muse who gave me the courage and calmed my stomach."

"Ah, dear little Muse," I sighed. "She is quite a mystery. There is no question she was a powerful source of inspiration, but…"

"But?"

"Was *she* the source of inspiration or did it come from within, from inside you and Wild Fingers and the others? I don't know. However, she did tell me one other thing before she left, something that I'm sure you will find interesting."

"What's that?"

"She said that she would become good friends with our baby."

"Well, what do you know. Maybe this child is destined for greatness."

Night Clinic Zebras

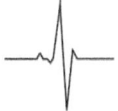

"LESS THAN TWO MONTHS TO GO AND I'LL FINALLY BE A real doctor," I announced as I walked through the door to the Night Clinic.

"I know, I know," Miss James answered, not even looking up from her desk. "Then, you can spend every night here at the Clinic, instead of two or three times a month."

"Dermatology, remember… Hawaii, beaches, sun," I replied, "a better, safer place to raise our daughter?"

"But, what about all the good you can do? These people love you. So many have said they wait for those nights you're working to come in."

"Yeah, everything that's creepy, strange, and bizarre manages to find its way to our Clinic. But, be reasonable for once…"

She raised an eyebrow at this request.

"…We'll have a new baby. My derm residency will be at a brand new, modern hospital, in a clean, safe part of town, and it will be regular hours. What have we here? The dregs of society, maggots, winos, addicts…"

"*People*," she said in a forceful voice, "people who have nothing else and nowhere to turn sometimes. How can you just turn your back and leave?"

She's right. Far too often I forget why I became a doctor. Still there's something to be said for a quality lifestyle and Dermatologists really do help their patients. Maybe, not in quite the same way…

"Enough discussion for one evening, let's get down to work," I announced.

"Oh, was that a 'discussion'? I thought it was an argument," she retorted.

I started to say something and stopped myself.

Let the pregnant lady have the last word.

"Any patients ready?"

She gave me a look that could have melted Antarctica and then her expression mellowed as she announced, "Marta Valdez, four years old, failure to thrive. She and her mother are in Room One."

"Thank you, dear, lovely Nurse," I answered, doing my best to be charming.

"Save it," was her reply.

I picked up the chart. Marta... four years old, twenty eight pounds, thirty four inches tall, well below normal parameters, no allergies...

I knocked and entered.

"Good evening, I'm Dr. Barnes," I said and extended my hand to greet Marta and her mother. "You must be Marta," I added as I shook the little girl's hand, "and you are Marta's mother?"

"Dora, Dora Weisel. I hope you can help us."

"I will certainly do my best," I replied. "Now can you tell me more about Marta, please?"

"Well, as I wrote on the history form, she's four and she just doesn't seem to be growing. She gets tired all the time; sometimes she's short of breath just from walking up the stairs. And, this evening, she had some blood when she went to the bathroom. That's why we came at this odd hour."

"I'm glad you brought her tonight, particularly if she is having bleeding. When did you first notice a problem?"

"Maybe six months ago. We went to the park and after playing for about fifteen minutes she came and sat down next to me. She said she felt tired. I know that by itself doesn't mean much, but she'd never done that before. She's always been the little whirlwind. I mean I could never keep up with her."

"Has she always been small?" I asked. I wasn't sure if Dora

could sense the concern that was growing inside me.

"Why, yes, but she doesn't seem to be growing much now."

I asked Marta if she hurt anywhere and she shook her head.

Small, but otherwise healthy appearing child tires easily and growth is stunted. Cardiac anomaly? Childhood cancer? Malabsorption? I started my exam. I examined her from head to toe. She had a small purplish skin lesion on her arm, probably an insignificant hemagioma.

Then I heard them, the bruits, everywhere, pounding in her chest and abdomen. What was that condition? The skin lesion, that insignificant hemagioma steered me to the diagnosis, a hopeless diagnosis for someone so young: Osler-Weber-Rendu, a syndrome with multiple arteriovenous malformations. I had no doubt, although I knew I'd need to send her to the Pediatric Oncology clinic for confirmation. I'd only read about this disease. I don't even know why I remembered such a rare illness.

She's awfully young to get this disease. Maybe it's something else. It doesn't really matter. Whatever it is, it's bad.

I looked at her chest X-Ray and labs and noted the abnormalities.

I steeled myself as I prepared to present all this information to a very worried mother.

"Ms. Weisel," I began, "it is very likely that Dora has a rare disease, a disease that is even rarer to be found in a child her age. I think she has this condition called Osler Weber Rendu. I know that means nothing to you. What it means is that as her blood circulates it goes through these things called Arteriovenous malformations. In doing so it bypasses the body's tissues and, as a result, those tissues and organs don't get their proper nutrition, like they are being starved. That's why she is so tired and that's why she isn't growing. Adults with this disease have finished growing and can compensate, but someone like her, well, to tell you the truth, I'm not sure what will happen."

"Are you sure about this, Dr. Barnes?" she wondered.

It's just an educated guess.

"I've only done a history and physical and a few labs and chest X-Ray, but the findings are pretty striking to me. But, to be sure she would need more testing, probably a CAT Scan or MRI to make a definite diagnosis. That's why I'm sending you to University Hospital, Dr. Katy Lenore. She's wonderful with the kids she treats, caring and brilliant. She's the smartest doctor I know."

"What should we do for now?"

I saw tears filling her eyes and then I saw Marta tugging on her mother's shirt.

"It's OK, Mommy. I'll work real hard to eat and grow and get better. I don't want you to cry," Marta said in a small, but determined voice.

Ms. Weisel dried her tears and picked up her little Marta. "I'm sure you will, my little darling and then we can come back and tell Dr. Barnes just how wrong he was."

She turned to me and shook my hand. I had to force myself to look into her eyes.

"I hope I'm wrong, truly I do, and I look forward to the day when you and Marta come back to tell me so."

I gave Ms. Weisel copies of my notes and the test results, and wished them well, and then went on to my next patient. Harry Wilcox, 29, abdominal pain and nausea for three years.

Harry Wilcox… Harry Wilcox, surely it can't be the same person. He should be back in Virginia.

Harry Wilcox is the name of a classmate of mine from high school, very popular, a three-letter man, football, basketball and track, and one of the biggest bullies I'd ever met. I always had assumed that he had gone on to great things. Surely this same Harry Wilcox wouldn't show up late at night in our little Clinic.

I knocked on the door and went in, and was greeted by Mr. Harry Wilcox, Class of 2003, Jefferson High School. We recognized each other immediately as he rose and held out his hand.

"Dr. Barnes, Dr. Barnes," he stated loudly, "I always knew

you'd end up as a doctor or astrophysicist or something intellectual. Still playing chess?"

"Not too much," I replied, "sick people keep me sort of busy."

I was doing my best to not show any animosity, but hatred that had been buried inside for years was starting to claw its way to the surface of my brain.

"What can I do for you," I asked, changing the subject. "What brought you into our quiet little night Clinic?"

He would not be deterred, however, as he went back to reminiscing.

"Remember the time we were playing Central for the division championship in basketball? We won on my last second shot from the corner. Anyway, you couldn't make it because someone had locked you in the janitor's closet. Did you ever figure out who did that?"

"Not definitely, but I'd always assumed it was you or one of your cronies. You know I almost died of dehydration."

"Really, that must have been terrible for you."

Quite the understatement. Locked in a closet on Friday and forgotten. At least there was a bucket. With every tortured minute, I vowed revenge. But, I've grown since then; revenge is such a petty thing. Or is it?

"Listen, Harry, I would love to sit and talk about ancient history, but you are not the only sick person here tonight. What can I do for you?"

"Well, Dr. Barnes, sort of rolls off the tongue, Doc...tor...Bar...nes, I've had episodes of abdominal pain and nausea off and on for about three years. I've been to doctor after doctor, specialists from Johns Hopkins to the Mayo Clinic, and nobody can figure it out. I heard from a friend of a friend that you moonlighted at this Clinic, so I figured why not go see my brilliant, intellectual former schoolmate. Maybe he can figure it out; maybe he knows me well enough to get to the root of the issue. And, here I am."

Now's my chance to get even, settle the score. Maybe serial enemas or placement of a thirty French foley catheter. Wait a minute, Doctor, don't forget Hippocrates. But, Hippocrates was never locked in a closet for three days.

"I would assume you've had a complete work up? You know, blood tests, X-Rays, GI endoscopy and such," I asked.

"You better believe it. Upper and lower GI's, CAT Scans, nuclear studies, I even had my gallbladder removed and I'm still sick."

"OK, Mr. Wilcox..."

"Harry, please call me Harry. After all, we are old friends."

"That is a matter of opinion. Let's keep it on a professional level, Mr. Wilcox. I guess I'll start with the basics. When did you first start having symptoms?"

Harry Wilcox breathed a deep sigh and then began his story.

"It was three years, one month, fourteen days, and three hours ago that I felt the first twinges of pain. I remember clearly because I had just finished a late dinner, fettuccini alfredo with shrimp, sautéed spinach, poppy seed rolls, Italian salad, and raspberry white chocolate cheesecake for dessert. It was at La Trattoria in Baltimore where I had just closed a business deal. Shortly after dinner, as I was sharing a few drinks with a young lady in my hotel room, and progressing quite well, if you get my drift, I was struck by waves of nausea, followed by intense pain in the middle of my abdomen, then I vomited about ten times, then more pain and finally, after about an hour I was better. Food poisoning, I figured. Of course, any thoughts of continuing my amorous ways went away with the buckets of puke, so I gave my companion a twenty and went to bed. It's been the same thing off and on for the last three years. Waves of nausea, aching sometimes intense pain, more nausea, vomiting, pain, and then it goes away."

"Tried taking any medication for these symptoms?" I queried.

"Advil, Pepto Bismol, Pepcid, Prilosec, Bentyl, Librax; none really help," Wilcox answered.

"Any particular food that triggers it, or stress, or anything you can think of that may be associated?"

He thought for a moment before answering. "I've noticed there is usually some sort of excitement before the symptoms commence. Gambling, or an impending female submission, or anything which causes a bit of mental strain."

Now it was my turn to think. "Do you get any headaches with these GI symptoms? Or any feeling that you are about to have an attack?"

He shook his head, "No, never have any headaches. It always starts with nausea first, then pain, then more nausea, and vomiting, usually."

I was beginning to get an idea, an unusual but not unheard of cause of abdominal symptoms, Abdominal Migraines, more common in children, but also found in adults. Treatment was a bit of a problem as there was no universally-accepted therapy.

"I'll be back in a minute," I said and I stepped out into the hall.

I hate to have to look things up on-the-fly like so many of the other residents, but…

I did a quick search for Abdominal Migraines and found very little which was helpful. There was one recommendation to use tricyclics and anti-anxiety meds. I went back to the Exam Room.

"Mr. Wilcox, I think I've found a medication that may help you. Take it twice a day, after breakfast and at bedtime. Come back and see me or your Primary Care Doctor in about two weeks."

I wrote out a prescription for Limbitrol DS and sent him on his way.

It's time for a nice case of the sniffles.

"New patient in Room Four, abdominal pain, rash, hair loss, diarrhea. I'm not sure what he's got, but he looks sick. Let me know as soon as you need an ambulance; I'm pretty sure you'll be sending him to the hospital."

"Serge Mostov, 58, no allergies, hypertension, c/o… hmm," I murmured and then I knocked and went into Room Four.

"Good evening, Mr. Mostov, what brings you in here tonight?"

"Didn't you read the forms, Dr.…, what is it?" he inquired squinting at my badge.

"Oh, I'm sorry, Dr. Barnes, it's Dr. Barnes and I did read the chart, but I like to hear it from the horse's mouth."

"Well, I'm no horse but I get your meaning," he replied.

Mr. Mostov had an eastern European accent. Russian, I thought. He definitely looked ill, skin had a gray pallor and I could see small clumps of hair on the floor.

Hypothyroid perhaps?

"When did your symptoms start, Mr. Mostov?"

"A few days ago. I went out for brunch, had my usual tea, a bagel with cream cheese, a bit of smoked salmon. That night I didn't feel well, so I only drank a bit of tea and went to bed. I've eaten nothing since and then I started with the hair falling out and diarrhea and pains."

Radiation?

"What do you do for a living, Mr. Mostov?"

"I'm in international trade. I expedite shipments of manufactured goods from Russia, Czech Republic, Turkey, all the eastern European countries. Here's my card."

Mostov Importing
PO Box 4005
New York, NY 10017

"You're a long way from New York," I observed.

"That's just my business address. I travel all over the country. I had a meeting here in town which is why I'm in your Clinic at this late hour."

"You aren't a spy are you, Mr. Mostov?" I wondered out loud. "Because your symptoms could be due to radiation poisoning."

He gave me a funny look and then clutched his stomach and moaned for about one minute and then he relaxed.

"That's how it has been for the last two days."

"Let me feel your pulse, please."

He held out his wrist and I put my fingers over the radial artery;

the pulse was present but definitely weak. I looked down at the chart. Vital signs were normal.

"Lay down on the table here so I can check you out," I requested.

There were sores in his mouth, which bled easily, and there was a slight conjunctival hemorrhage, which I hadn't noticed when I first walked in the room. His abdomen was diffusely tender and there was frank blood in his rectum. I checked his blood pressure and it was 80/45 and heart rate was 115.

"If I were to bet, Mr. Mostov, you have been poisoned. We've called an ambulance to take you to the hospital. I'll also call to let Dr. Astor in the ICU know what's going on. Do you have any family? Because you should call them."

"Is it that bad, Dr. Barnes?"

"I think it's worse."

"Then, please, call this number from the pay phone which is down the block and tell the person who answers your suspicions. First give them this number: 545-234-323. You have my permission. They will know what to do. And, now I will leave you."

But, the ambulance is on its way. If you leave I am sure you won't survive twenty four hours."

"And if I go in your ambulance, how long will I survive? Perhaps twenty five hours? I have unfinished business to attend to. I thank for your time, Dr. Barnes. For your own safety, please leave no record of my visit here. Good evening and thank you again."

He picked up his coat and walked out. I called the number on the card he had given me and reached the Russian Embassy. I delivered his message, they thanked me and I hung up. I stayed in the shadows as I made my way back to the Clinic, just in case.

I reached the Clinic entrance unseen. As I pulled the door open I heard a noise, like hoof beats on a cobblestone road. I turned and saw two zebras run by. I walked back into the Clinic shaking my head.

Not surprised.

"Where'd you go?" Miss James queried. "Four patients are waiting."

"Simple things, I hope," I answered, ignoring her question.

"Back pain in One, swollen hand in Two, fever in Three and 'black penis' in Four."

"Really?"

"That's what he put down. His vitals are normal, but I didn't examine his chief complaint. You men are so funny about down there."

"Shouldn't we be? I think I'll save 'The Black Penis' for last," I remarked as I picked up the chart to Room One.

Michael Smoots, 38, back pain for four hours, no medical problems, normal vital signs.

With any luck a shot of morphine and follow up at the Ortho Clinic will do the trick.

I did my usual knocking and went in. I found Mr. Smoots stretched out on the exam table, staring at the ceiling. He was pale and from the doorway I could see tiny red spots covering his body.

Here we go again.

"Mr. Smoots, I'm Dr. Barnes. What seems to be the problem?"

"The problem? You're a doctor; look at me. My back feels like someone stuck it with a cattle prod and now my toes are going numb and I may have had an accident while laying here."

"And all this just started four hours ago? What about all those red spots?"

"They just appeared while I've been laying here. What's going on, Dr. Barnes? I feel like I'm about to die."

"I'm not going to let that happen, Mr. Smoots, but we need to get you to the hospital."

I pushed the intercom button, a device I hated and rarely used because it broadcast all over the Clinic.

"Miss James, I need you, now."

The door promptly opened and my able assistant appeared.

We need an ambulance, I need an IV set up, and I need some

antibiotics, Rocephin, everything five minutes ago."

She didn't ask any questions as I applied a tourniquet to my patient's arm and started an 18 g IV in the antecubital area. I opened up the fluids and pushed the Rocephin the moment Miss James put it in my hand.

"What is it, Dr. Barnes?"

"Most likely Meningococcal meningitis, but it could be a spinal cord abscess or tumor. Whatever it is, it's an emergency which needs more treatment than we can provide here."

"Ambulance will be here in two minutes."

"Good, good. Mr. Smoots, are you OK?"

"I've developed a terrible headache and the numbness is worse."

"Just hang in there. The ambulance is here. You'll be up dancing in no time."

I saw him visibly wince at my words and then I realized why. Michael Smoots, was a dancer and choreographer for City Center Dance. He was famous. I saw him on television and he'd even done a stint on Broadway in "Pippen."

They loaded him on the stretcher as I silently berated myself for my lack of insight.

"Take good care of him, boys," I exhorted the ambulance attendants.

And they wheeled him away into the night.

I looked at my watch, 3:34.

This night is never going to end.

Room Two, John Hedrick, 41, swollen hand for three days, no fever, history of Type I Diabetes, no allergies. I paused for a moment and then forged ahead, knocked, and greeted Mr. Hedrick.

"Good evening Mr…" before I could finish I was welcomed by a man waving one of those big fake hands with the index finger sticking up shouting "We're Number One," most commonly seen at sporting events.

"Dr. Barnes, he's our man, if he can't do it nobody can, Rah," he shouted jumping up and down.

He was wearing the local football team's red and white colors with Mustangs plastered across his chest, his face was painted red on one side and white on the other.

"I don't take care of delusional patients," I began. "Our Mustangs haven't come close to finding their way out of the cellar for what is it? Eight years?"

"But, we're poised for the big break out," he cheered.

"Uh, Mr. Hedrick, I wish I could humor you in your fantasies, but I have a very sick man dying from a black penis waiting to be seen. Is there something I can help you with?"

"Like I wrote on the paper, I've got a swollen hand."

"I see that, very clever."

"It's this hand, Dr. Barnes," and he held out his left hand which really was swollen and slightly bluish.

I cradled his hand in mine and felt for the radial pulse, which was present and bounding. He winced slightly even though I grabbed his hand ever so gently.

"How long has this been swollen and tender?" I asked.

"Started four days ago at ten in the morning. I was loading crates on a truck when I felt a twinge in my finger..."

"Which finger?"

"The middle finger, right here." He held up his middle finger and pointed to the area of the metacarpal-phalangeal joint. It was definitely swollen and hot.

Gout? The start of Rheumatoid Arthritis? This was going to take more testing than we could do at our Clinic.

"Have you had any fever?"

"Just in my hand."

"I'm not sure what it is. It could be gout or some type of arthritis. I don't think it's any infection. We'll check some blood tests and do an X-Ray and then we'll know more."

"Thank you, Dr. Barnes," Mr. Hedrick answered.

I always like polite patients.

Miss James will be in here to take your blood and get the X-Rays done, and then I'll be back.

I went back to the break room before tackling "The Black Penis." I opened the back and stood in the alley, hearing the hoof beats again. Like before I saw zebras run by, only this time there were four. I watched until they faded from site and then I took a deep breath and marched to Room Four where "The Black Penis" was waiting.

Elmore Doddington, 29, no previous medical problems, complaining of penis turning black for eleven hours.

Not surprised he didn't wait too long before coming in. Miss James is right about men and their penises.

I knocked loudly, waited a few seconds, and then forged ahead.

"Good evening, Mr. Doddington, what is the problem you are having?"

"My problem? Just look at this."

He pulled the paper sheet away that was covering his groin area and revealed his private parts which were, just as reported, black, but also swollen and starting to rot.

"How did this start?"

"I think it was this afternoon. I was sitting in the park, feeding the ducks, like I always do in the morning. I had finished tossing bread crumbs when I sensed the presence of someone or something sitting next to me and then I felt a sharp pain in the tip of my penis; I thought it was a bug bite. Of course, I couldn't just pull my pants down and check right there, so I dumped out the last few bread crumbs and went behind the bushes, just to take a quick look.

"Well, there was a tiny black spot on the end which was painful. Spider bite was my first thought. But, I didn't find a spider. Anyway, the black spot started to grow. That was when I figured it out."

"What did you figure out?" I asked.

"Who or should I say *what* had bitten me. Actually it was staring me in the face the whole time: 'Invisible Gay Zombies from the

Underworld.' "

"Excuse me?" I stumbled over my words.

"It's right here," and he held up a copy of the Daily Encounter, a tabloid paper well known for over embellished reporting.

"Invisible Gay Zombies Invade Our World and Accost Teenager, Fifteen Year Old Boy is in Catatonic State"

I glanced through the article which touched on a boy named Chase, the fifteen-year-old who had been assaulted, but never saw his assailant. The boy then turned into a "Zombie" which in his case meant he entered a catatonic-like state, unresponsive to any stimulus, eyes staring blankly at the distance.

I wonder where the Underworld comes into play.

Mr. Doddington continued, as if he'd read my mind, "They must be from the Underworld because they come out of the sewers. And, there's a manhole cover not more than twenty feet from where I was sitting in the park. I'm sure I heard the sound of that cover being replaced and then, Whammo, my penis starts to turn black and before the day is out I'll be a Zombie, nothing but rotting flesh and malevolence."

I stared at my patient and the look on my face must not have instilled any confidence.

"If you don't believe *me*, then how do *you* explain my symptoms?"

"Necrotizing infection secondary to Strep..."

"With no fever, normal vital signs, and no pain. I work as a nurse; I have a bit of medical knowledge."

"You certainly are correct; there should be some systemic signs of infection if this is truly a necrotizing infection."

Definitely one of the more bizarre conditions I've ever encountered. Maybe he stuck his privates into a vise or zapped it with a cattle prod. What to do? What to do?

An idea popped into my head.

Won't cause any harm and I can always send him to the hospital.

"Mr. Doddington, I'm afraid Zombies are a bit out of my field of expertise. I think I skipped that lecture; but I do know someone who can help. She's an expert in Zombies and voodoo and such and she lives only a short distance away."

"Well, you better get her here fast, because in forty three minutes and eighteen seconds the zombification process will become irreversible.

I nodded my head as if I understood completely. In reality I had no idea what he was talking about. I have to admit the finer points of Zombies have not been a part of my medical studies and I've never watched *Walking Dead*.

I searched on the computer for "Voodooweightloss.com" specifically looking for Madame Marie, Voodoo High Priestess.

If anyone can help me with a Zombie problem, it's her.

Miss James saw me clicking through the pages.

"Another voodoo problem?"

"Zombie," I corrected her.

"I have Madame Marie on speed dial," and she stooped over to help me, giving me an eyeful of her cleavage in the process.

Once a letch, always a letch.

"Good evening, Madame? This is Nurse James. Oh, I'm fine. Yes, the spell worked perfectly... thank you... Dr. Barnes over here at the Night Clinic wants to talk to you."

"Here you go," and she handed me her phone. I gave her a look of surprise as I took the phone.

"Good evening, Madame. How's the weight loss business? I'm sorry, but we've got a bit of an emergency over here... No, not really voodoo, at least I don't think so... It's a Zombie problem... almost twelve hours... eleven hours and forty minutes give or take a few seconds... You'll be right over... thanks."

I turned to Miss James. "She's on her way, she has to stop and pick up a chicken foot and said that the victim needs to have a valuable personal item and $225 cash."

"Good old Madame Marie," Miss James commented.

"Oh and why do you have her number listed with your contacts?" I wondered.

Miss James looked up at the ceiling, "I hope she gets here soon," she added.

"Don't try to change the subject. Why does a nurse for this Clinic have a voodoo high priestess on speed dial, and what was all that talk about a spell?"

"Come, come, Dr. Barnes, with everything that has happened since you've been working here? Besides Madame, I've also got a Priest, a Rabbi, a Buddhist Monk, a Hindu Shaman, the FBI, the CIA, the Fire Department, Animal Control, the Police Department, the Sheriff's Office, and Ghostbusters on my contact list."

While we waited for the Voodoo High Priestess to arrive I went back to Room Three to finish up with Mr. Hedrick. His X-rays revealed bony destruction involving the third finger.

I went back to Room Three.

"Mr. Hedrick," I began, "it looks like you have some sort of infection or inflammation involving the bones of your left hand."

I re-examined his hand and his forearm. There was an area of swelling above his elbow, which was also tender.

"Have you been scratched or bitten by a cat recently?"

"Not that I remember," he replied.

"Any exposure to tuberculosis?"

"No. Nothing unusual has happened. I've done nothing but go to work, eat, and lay on the beach."

"Lay on the beach? That could be the answer," I decided. "I think you have some unusual form of infection, a rare type of bacteria, sort of like tuberculosis, but not exactly. Unfortunately, we don't have the means to test for it here. I'm going to write you out a prescription and I think you should go over to the hospital ER. I don't think we'll need an ambulance, but I will call them and tell them you're on your way."

"Which hospital?" he asked

"University. I think if they'll be able to fix you up."

We sent him on his way and called the University ER and told them to expect his visit.

About a minute later the sound of the bell out front chimed, ringing over and over as someone was banging it repeatedly.

"Some people can't read," I muttered referring to our sign, which said: *Please ring the bell one time for service.*

The bell kept ringing and when I arrived at the reception desk I found a short, thin, dark-skinned woman pounding away. She was dressed in a colorful wraparound dress and had a matching scarf on her head. She was carrying a canvas bag.

"Good morning, Dr. Barnes. I'm Madame Marie," and she held out her hand. "Now, take me to our poor Zombie."

She had a definite Caribbean accent, was about five foot nothing, very white teeth, except for a single gold tooth in the front, and she smelled of flowers.

Reminds me of Dr. Adams.

I led our High Priestess to Room Four and introduced her to Mr. Doddington. She stared him up and down, and then opened her bag and started putting things on the counter: a small doll which looked like our victim, a metal plate with some coal on it, a string of garlic, and two raw bird's feet one larger than the other.

"Now, young man. I'll need a valuable personal item and $225."

"That seems a bit steep and I didn't bring anything of value with me."

"OK, Ok, young man," she responded as she bounced up and down on her heels. "But, your pecker is about to fall off and in thirteen minutes you will be entering the irreversible state of Zombification. It's your choice. You have a very nice ring on your right hand, only fourteen-carat gold, but at least it has a real diamond, SI2, H color, good cut. That will suffice for our purposes."

Doddington peaked under his gown and then pulled the ring off his finger and handed it to Madame along with $225 he pulled from his wallet.

"One more business item before I get to work. Which raw bird's foot would you like? We have the standard raw chicken foot, which will return you to your original state and size. Or, we have the ostrich foot, which will provide significant enhancements for an additional $75."

Doddington looked a little perplexed.

I interjected, "If I understand Madame Marie correctly, you may have a Ballpark Frank for $225 or a Hebrew National Knockwurst for $300."

"I guess I'm not very hungry, so Ballpark please," he decided.

Madame shrugged her shoulders, took his money and his ring, and lit a match to the coals which were glowing hot in about a minute. She threw the ring in with coals and then tied a sort of athletic supporter around Doddington's waist.

Next she poured all the hot coals but one, along with the melted ring and the chicken's foot, sans one toe, into the athletic supporter and waved the lone chicken toe and the doll over his waist. She chanted a few incoherent words and danced around the table, holding the coal in her hand.

The smell of burning flesh, from Madame's hand and Doddington's necrotic penis, filled the room as the lights went out and the room took on an unworldly eeriness as the only illumination came from the glowing coal in the High Priestess' hand.

Finally, Madame Marie thrust her hand into the athletic supporter and there was a scream from the High Priestess, I think. The lights came on and the burning smell vanished.

I looked at the clock, one minute four seconds to spare. My patient looked under his gown and took off the athletic supporter.

"Looks good as new," he reported. He pulled out his ring, which was truly looking sparkling and brand new. "Everything else also is better."

"Let me check the results, just for my documentation," I requested.

Sure enough he had a normal appearing penis, pink and healthy.

Madame Marie held up her hand which was free of any burn or scar. She fastened the chicken toe to a leather cord and handed it to our patient. The toe looked like it had been cooked.

"Wear this around your neck for at least six months, night and day, even in the shower or bath. It will keep those Invisible Gay Zombies from making a return visit.

"And you, Dr. Barnes, this clinic is also vulnerable. For $75 I'll leave the ostrich foot here to ward off any evil interlopers."

I looked at the big ostrich foot and then handed it back to the High Priestess.

"Without a steady stream of 'evil interlopers' this clinic wouldn't have any reason to stay open," I informed her, "so you may keep it. Save it for someone who really needs it."

Miss James and I escorted Madame Marie and Mr. Doddington out of the Clinic and watched as they went their separate ways. The clinic was empty now and the sun was just peaking out of the horizon in the east.

"How did you know?" Miss James asked.

"How did I know what?"

"About the Zombies? That Mr. Doddington didn't have some sort of dreaded disease that was about to kill him?"

"I didn't. All I knew was that I'd never heard of any disease which caused only necrosis of the penis. Usually it's quite the opposite. I've seen patients come in with terrible infections in the groin area which, after proper investigation, started from a bite on the penis. In every one of those cases, the penis, for whatever reason, is spared the tissue necrosis. I guess God made the penis almost indestructible."

"I'm glad," she answered. "But, maybe you should have kept that ostrich foot. Madame Marie did promise that it could bring significant enhancement."

"I've never had any complaints," I remarked.

At that moment I heard hoof beats pounding on the pavement. A few moments later a herd of zebras ran in front of the clinic, their stripes lighting up pink and yellow in the soft light of the rising sun.

"Back to normal, I guess," we said in unison.

NIGHT CLINIC RAVEN

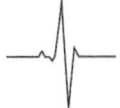

"I DON'T LIKE THE LOOKS OF THIS," I SAID AS I WALKED into the Clinic. I looked up and saw a large black bird perched on the sign with the big red cross which hung above our entrance. Then I let my gaze travel up to the early evening sky, and I saw the full moon and murmured to myself, "It's going to be a long night."

"Did you see that bird perched outside our Clinic?" I asked Miss James as she looked up from the desk where she had stowed her monstrous purse.

"No, I guess not," she answered. "I hurried in without taking any notice so I wouldn't be late."

"Well, it's got to be the biggest crow ever. Black feathers, black feet, black beak, all outlined by a full moon. And, I think it had devilish red eyes. A fiendish bird and a full moon? One or the other and I'd say we were in for a long night, but the two together spells disaster of Biblical proportion. I'm sure it won't be sore throats and sprained ankles all night."

Miss James stuck her head outside. The sun was almost settled down in the west and the full moon had taken its place commanding the dusk. She stood opposite the sign which swayed gently back and forth in the light breeze.

"It's funny how it just sits there, perched quietly, almost serene in the moonlight. It's a raven, you know, like a crow, but solitary," she observed.

"It all seems very Poe-ish to me, 'quoth the raven, nevermore.' I never did understand that poem."

I turned to my right and felt a sharp twinge of pain in my side.

Miss James noticed me wincing as the pain shot into my thigh.

"Dr. Barnes, are you alright? For a moment you turned white as a ghost."

I caught my breath and slowly straightened up. "Yes, yes, I don't know what that was. I guess I just turned too suddenly and had some sort of muscle spasm. But it still hurts. I guess I'll go sit down for a minute while you get the first patients ready.

"Good idea, Doctor," she agreed with me for once.

Full moon, ravens, talk of turning white like a ghost. Maybe I should call Dr. Maxim to cover for me and take the night off. Two bad omens I can handle, but three surely means this night will never end.

I glanced outside and saw that the Raven was still perched above our door. I felt a tap on my shoulder as Miss James beckoned me back inside to start our shift.

"We should close the Clinic tonight," I decided. "I've got a bad feeling."

"Don't be silly," she chided me and then she went outside and shoed the black bird away. "See, it's gone."

"Not really," I replied as the Raven returned and settled once again on top of our sign.

"It's just a bird. There's a child with a fever and sore throat in Room One," she announced.

"Good, something easy for a change," I said and we walked back towards the Exam Rooms together.

"You're walking sort of bent over," Miss James noticed. "Something wrong?"

"I've got this soreness in my right side, seems to hurt more if I stand up straight. Maybe I pulled a muscle running this morning."

I picked up the chart outside the door of Exam Room One. Amber Lynn, 2 years old, sore throat and cough for two days, temp 101, otherwise healthy.

A nice straightforward five-minute visit.

"Good evening, I'm Dr. Barnes, and this must be Amber," I began my usual introduction and held out my hand to Amber's mother.

We went through the brief history and I checked the little girl's throat and listened to her chest. As I was writing out a prescription and instructions for Amber's now relieved Mother, I heard a loud crash and shouting from the waiting room.

"Wait here," I instructed and went out to see what had caused all the commotion.

I walked quickly out to the waiting room, almost colliding with Miss James and her big belly, and arrived at the lobby just in time to see two young men in colorful leather jackets and jeans at each other's throats.

One of the combatants gained the upper hand and pulled his adversary up with his arm wrapped around his neck. I started towards them.

"You two monsters take your differences outside. You know the 'rules,' this Clinic is safe…"

"…for what this asshole did, there is no safe place." And he pulled out a blade and slashed it across his opponent's neck. I raced to the victim's side, ignoring the now very intense pain in my right side.

"Nobody's going to bleed to death in my Clinic," I shouted, pushing his attacker away.

"You don't get involved, Doc. He deserves to die for what he did to my little sister," the attacker screamed back. "You stay away from him. Just let him bleed. I'm warning you…"

I ignored this warning as I pulled off my shirt and held pressure over the deep neck wound, pushing my fingers into the depths of his neck to stem the blood flow, putting direct pressure over what I hoped was not his carotid artery. The fountain of blood slowed to a trickle as I cradled the victim's head.

"I warned you," said a voice behind me.

I felt a sharp pain just above my belly button and then looked up at my attacker as he pulled his knife out of my abdomen. My head started to spin as I heard a vaguely familiar musical jingle in the background. I looked up and saw the Raven settling on the light above me. Then I saw the Raven open its mouth, as if to speak, and I remember eagerly anticipating its words… but there was only silence as everything went black.

After some unknown period of time, the dark dissolved and a refined, sophisticated, slightly British voice began:

"You should feel lucky, you know. You should be dead, but somehow somebody snatched you from the abyss, at least for a moment."

I opened my eyes and saw the Raven. I tried to reach up and grab him; I wanted to strangle the life out of him. I wasn't sure why I hated him so, but in my mind he was the embodiment of all the evil I had ever known. My arms wouldn't move.

"You should hate me, you are right to hate me, but you don't completely understand the whys and wherefores. I'm sorry, that's redundant."

A learned Raven?

"Oh, don't try to answer. Your arms are tied down and you've got a tube in your throat so you can't talk. You know the kind, an ET tube, you're on a ventilator, life support. It's all that stands between you and an eternity with the likes of me. As a matter of fact, you've got tubes coming out of most of your body orifices. Therefore, just blink your eyes if you understand me."

I tried to move but I couldn't. I opened my mouth to scream at that vile bird, but there was only silence. I blinked my eyes twice.

"Once is enough. You don't need to shout. I know what you're thinking. What does a raven have to do with you or your precious Night Clinic or anything at all? You're a smart doctor; you should know. You have this notion that I am wicked, but we ravens are not evil harbingers of ill will. Truly, we are one of god's chosen messengers, like angels. Oh, you don't believe me? Don't take my word for it, just look in the Bible. Who did God choose to feed the prophet Elijah? Ravens. And who did Noah first send out from the Ark to 'test the waters'? A raven. So don't go carrying on about evil and the dark side of humanity. You don't have to say it; these thoughts fill your head. Sometimes I wish Edgar Allen Poe had never been born."

I wished the Raven would stop his incessant chatter, but I was helpless. All I could do was lay there and listen.

I must be in a hospital on a ventilator, which means the Raven is correct that I can't talk. Maybe, I died and this is really Hell. Is this my fate? To be trapped for Eternity listening to the rantings of a deranged crow?

"Crow, did you call me a crow? Why, I've never been so insulted. Crows are vicious and petty. Just look at what a group of them is called: a Murder. How appropriate. Every time I see one of those little flying rats I'd like to **murder it**. But, ravens, we are a different breed, the most noble of all birds. Solitary, thoughtful, central to such a variety of myth and legend. Why, it was the ravens of London Tower that maintained the British Empire. The ravens are part of the great Norse god, King Odin. So, please don't offend me by calling me a crow."

His voice had grown loud and pierced my brain, but I guess he realized how shrill he had become and settled down.

"Now, where were we? Ah, yes, the nobility of the raven, a favorite topic of mine. But, enough about me, let us talk about you. Rather, I will talk, you listen. You really do listen very well, although I suppose you don't have a choice."

There was a sigh and then he continued. "I wish all doctors were such good listeners. It's the ability to listen and hear what their patients are saying that makes a doctor a truly skilled healer. But, are you really a good doctor? Are you even a good person? You think you performed a brave and righteous act when you thrust your fingers into that dying boy's neck wound and saved his life, but was it in fact righteous? Do you know what he did to provoke such an attack? I'm sure you remember his assailant shouting about his sister, his baby sister, his nine-year-old baby sister who had just been brutally raped and then mutilated by the monster you saved. Does that make you feel noble? Don't try to answer. And, closing your eyes tightly won't make the truth go away. That beast deserved to suffer, deserved to die. Is it wrong for a brother to take vengeance on the person who attacked his sister and left her scarred beyond all hope for life? However, you did not know, you could not have known. And, if you had known the truth, if you had witnessed the atrocity, would you have been in such a hurry to save that boy?

"Your eyes plead ignorance, while your soul is in turmoil. But, there is no amount of penance which can undo such damage. Maybe, just maybe, you were right, you should have saved him. It's your job, you took an oath to treat the sick and injured to the best of your ability. It isn't *your* place to sit in judgment. But, tell me, are doctors exempt from simple human decency?

"Let us forget about your attacker and his victim for now. Let us look at something closer to you, the lovely, decent, and resourceful Miss James. She has almost molded you into an acceptable human being; one with a true conscience and respect for others. She drew you away from your shallow dreams and brought you into a bizarre world filled with society's outcasts, rejects and downtrodden. She faces each day with a smile and a helping hand not because it is a job, but because she cares about every drunk, junkie, and schizo that wanders into her clinic. CAN YOU SAY THE SAME?"

The Raven paused from his soliloquy for a moment and took a deep breath.

"I'm sorry I raised my voice. You, Dr. Barnes, you would escape from the Night Clinic in a moment if she would agree to join you and, now that you've suffered this terrible injury, she just might do that, just for you. But, can you ever truly escape? Your past will be with you. Yes, I know; I know all about a lazy, abusive, alcoholic father who cast his son out when the boy was barely fifteen. I know about this boy who survived on streets not unlike those which surround the Night Clinic, who lived by his wits, managed to go to school, worked every sort of odd job, and maintained an equilibrium that carried him to scholarships, then to one of our finest universities and, finally, medical school, all the while vowing to never return to the poverty of his childhood days.

"There is, however, a demon lurking in the shadows. Guilt. We all must deal with our guilt. Dermatology in Hawaii is as far from the Night Clinic as you could go, and the prospect of a soft life lounging on the beach unchained the guilt from the depths of your being and brought it to the surface where, eventually, it would have torn you apart. However, the presence of Miss James stifled your guilt while allowing you to rationalize your decision to stay at the Clinic. You say it's for her, but truly it's your guilt which keeps you surrounded by winos and hookers. I tell you the truth: if you were to try to leave this sordid world behind and abandon those members of society who most need your help, this guilt would devour you. Oh, you would surely feign happiness, drive around in your big, shiny Mercedes or BMW or Lexus, live in a big house on the beach, but underneath guilt would be gnawing away, scratching and tearing at your soul, never allowing you a moment's rest. Maybe it would have been a little thing like insomnia or something worse like uncontrollable fits of anger, or infidelity, but it would have been something. And then, because of this guilt, booze or pills or worse would have consumed you and, in the end, you would have ended up in exactly the same place you are now, except without hope.

"Oh, I've offended you, I'm sorry. Truth is always a burden and facing the truth within us is an even greater weight to shoulder, a weight which suffocates. That sounds very profound, doesn't it? 'Truth is always a burden, truth suffocates.' But it's just drivel, no, it's worse than drivel, it's foolish nonsense which deceives. It is running from the truth which creates the burden. However, admitting that there is truth and accepting it brings freedom, and freedom releases us from the troubles of this world. Well, maybe not us, at least not me, after all, I'm just an eloquent black bird. But, humanity is crushed by its refusal to face truth or even admit that there is such a thing as absolute truth in this world. And, what is this truth? Just three things: you are born, you struggle for a brief period of time, and you die, and on the day an individual accepts the reality of this truth, real freedom begins.

"I'm sorry, I've wandered off into the world of philosophy. I'll get off the soapbox and, let us see, where were we? Oh, yes, Miss James.

"She's your savior, you know. I know it's not a pretty picture, but look at what you were before she came into your life. A heartless womanizer, studying the intellectual side of medicine, but with no soul or true compassion. Intelligence and hard work may carry you a long way in the medical arts, but without a large dose of kindness and concern for others you could never be a true healer. Miss James, surrounded by the deprivation she lives with and fights on a daily basis in the clinic, opened your eyes to this world you knew all too well; one you had buried away deep in the recesses of your brain and hoped to escape forever. It was Miss James who guided you and showed you the true meaning of responsibility, compassion and, in the end, love. It's why you are lying here now instead of being safely ensconced in that cushy job treating annoying itches on the buttocks of fat, wealthy socialites."

I had been listening to his speech quietly, my eyes closed, each word boring into my brain, but now I wanted to answer him, tell him how right he was, but also how wrong.

He knows what's in your head; you don't have to tell him.

I opened my eyes. I wanted to speak to him and tell him, but he was gone. For a brief moment I heard the steady beeping of monitors and the whoosh of the ventilator, but these noises faded as reality receded and everything went black.

After a time, the black began to withdraw as streaks of light poked out from the edges of emptiness until I saw the silhouette of the Raven perched above me.

"I hope you had a peaceful respite," he began, "but, I see that was not the case. Perhaps I will be able to put your mind at ease. How can I do that? Surely you don't blame me for the turmoil you feel. I am not the one who stabbed you; I did not make you sick or harm you in any way. I did not suffer poverty and deprivation with you. I am only here now, a messenger to help, to bring peace to a tired soul, perhaps eternal peace. Death? Perhaps, but perhaps not. I know you've wondered about death over the years, pondered, searched, and even glimpsed a taste of what may come after one's breathing ceases, the heart beats its last, the brain becomes quiet. Is it the beautiful Garden? Is it complete and total nothingness? Is it anything? Here, let me show you, let me take you."

The Raven spread its wings and started to beat the air ever so slowly. It hovered above its perch for a moment and then moved closer, drawing me out of my bed and carrying me away. The wind raced past, bringing a delightful relief from the chaos in my soul. A patch of green began to grow in the distance, then that green space was split by a river of blue. Bits of color grew into radiant collages as flowers appeared and we stopped. The Raven, gently holding me aloft, hovered over the Garden. Not just any garden, *The Garden*. The exact garden that took Jewel and her mother; the same Garden I'd thought about almost every night since that fateful day. Here it was again and here I had a second chance. I knew what waited for me in that place: Peace. Peace and Eternal Happiness.

"It's yours, if you wish. Choose. You know what waits for you here in the Garden. Or, you may choose an unknown future. But, you must make a choice. You're a doctor. Every day you make life and death decisions. Now it's your own life. Choose."

Sick children, injured teens, hopeless diseases, death and destruction weighed on my head and then I saw the Garden, beautiful, peaceful, serene.

Is there any choice?

I reached down and tried to grab a branch to pull myself down, down into the Garden and away from the Raven. I had almost touched the top of one of the trees when the Raven left me and settled on a nearby tree branch and fixed his stare upon me.

"CHOOSE," he screamed.

And, above me, I saw the Goddess of the Night and Captain

Surgery and the Dragon and Caleb and so many others shouting at me, begging for me to come back, to help them, to ease their suffering, and I pulled my hand back. Below was Jewel beckoning, mouthing, "It's OK."

I heard the screams of a woman in labor, Miss James suffering for our child, for me, and then a final blood curdling scream, and then crying, first soft and then louder: the cries of a baby and her father.

"NO," I screamed as I ripped the endotracheal tube out of my throat and sat up in my hospital bed screaming, "NO, NO, NO."

Arms reached against my shoulders and held me down as I opened my eyes and saw Miss James, dear Miss James, and I felt her hand on mine. I settled back, comforted by the soothing, steady beeps of the EKG and pulse oximeter, and her sweet sweet voice.

"It's OK, Doctor, It's OK."

"I'm thirsty," I croaked out. "I won't need that tube anymore."

I felt the cold plastic of an oxygen mask settle on my face as I lay back and fell asleep to the lullaby of the ICU.

The Raven was gone.

I awoke to the caresses of Miss James stroking my cheek with her soft hand.

"You're looking much better, I must say. You've been through quite an ordeal. Did you know that besides being brutally stabbed while attempting to save a young man's life, you also had a ruptured appendix. It was all Captain Surgery could do to stem the bleeding and clean up all the infection. And then, despite the Captain's efforts, you've been on seven drips, suffered through ARDS, Renal failure, and shock liver. I don't know what was going on in your head, but your behavior was a little bit bizarre. They had to keep you tied down most of the time and you seemed to be staring at something, even though I don't think you saw any of *us* hovering over you. All I can say is that it's a good thing you're young and strong. At least it looks like you'll be around to see your daughter come into this world."

"Daughter? A baby girl?" My eyes lit up and I'm sure a big smile crept onto my face. "Wonderful... I'm glad," I murmured as I sank deeper into my bed.

"Now, my dear Miss James," I added, "do you think you can get me a rack of ribs from Louie's... and some cole slaw?"

Two weeks later I was back on my feet and made my return visit to the Night Clinic.

I walked towards the front entrance and saw the Raven perched on the sign above the door. Its gaze almost burned a hole in me as I walked by. I stopped in the doorway, turned, and smiled at my black benefactor and tormenter. Its beak opened as if it was going to address me, but then it smiled, closed its mouth, and I watched as it spread its wings and flew away.

Night Clinic Wedding

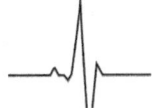

"I DON'T KNOW WHY WE'RE GETTING MARRIED HERE AT the Clinic. We could have had the Grand Ballroom at the Hilton for nothing. With our luck, the preacher will probably get mugged on his way here," I commented to my expectant betrothed. "And I still think we should have waited until you delivered. A couple of weeks wouldn't have changed anything."

Miss James gave me a look which said, "We've been through this a million times, don't bother me anymore." And then she spoke, "I do not want to have my daughter called a bastard, even for a few weeks."

"I know, I know," was all I could say. "It won't be much of a honeymoon," I muttered under my breath.

"Did you say something?"

"I said I hope Curley and Cupcake can still carry a tune," I replied loudly.

"Uh huh. Oh, here's my mother. I'll see you shortly."

"OK, lovely nurse," I replied as Miss James met her mother outside the Exam Room I was using to get dressed. "Wait, wait, I need you to help me tie this…" my voice trailed off as she vanished, "… bowtie."

I'm in trouble now. Where's that card with the step-by-step instructions.

I wrapped the black strap around my neck, crossed and folded just like in the diagram and… nothing, at least nothing that resembled a bowtie.

Whoever invented ties hated the human male; probably the same per-

son who invented high heels, some sort of equal opportunity tormenter.

I fixed my cummerbund and made one more effort to tie the bowtie, once again without success; I looked out at the arriving guests. I saw Daniel arrive with the Cichellos, faithful mutt, Becky, at his side, and motioned for him to come over.

"You look pretty spiffy," I pointed out. "Everything OK at your new digs?"

"Can't complain, three meals a day, warm place to sleep, cable TV," he answered.

"Good, good," I said. "Listen, can you do me a big favor? We've got about an hour until this shindig starts. Do you think you can run over to the thrift shop and see if they've got a black bowtie, one that's already tied? Here's twenty bucks, keep whatever you don't spend. And remember, pay for the tie, don't steal it."

"Sure thing, Dr. Barnes."

He and Becky ran out the door to Aaron's Thrift and Smoke Shop; I threw the troublesome bowtie in the trash. Once again, I peeked out into the Clinic waiting area, which now was a makeshift wedding chapel, and saw guests milling about. Mona "I'm a wedding consultant, not a planner" Avery was adjusting flowers on the crude altar which had been erected at one end of the waiting room. She turned around and watched as our guests filed in and made their way to their seats or chatted with each other. Mona's eyes grew wider and wider as this bizarre assortment of visitors arrived.

First there was Mrs. Cichello with Andrew, then Crystal Blue and the Wicked Queen, each dressed in spandex body suits, followed by the seven dwarfs from the Enchanted Emporium. A few seconds later Evella, Goddess of the Night, arrived, dressed in bright blue fishnet instead of her usual black. She took a seat near the front next to Caleb, who was sitting with his ever-present sketchpad and colored pencils. Policemen, winos, addicts, hookers and some who just looked curious passed through the doors and took seats near the back. I heard the familiar, "Da, da, da, daaa..." chiming as Captain Surgery and Dr. Cloud alighted outside the door and took their seats close to the front. The massive figure of Roachman with Super Rat perched on his shoulder burst through the doors and marched to the front, taking a seat in the second row. I suppose it was all too much for our wedding planner, all these curious, odd and extraordinary folks we called friends, because I saw Mona sneak out the back. We never heard from her again.

I felt a pull on the tails of my tux and turned around to see Daniel, waving the bowtie in front of me.

"Thanks, kid," I said. "Uh, you can stop waving it, I see that you were successful."

"I'm trying to get it to dry," he replied. "They only had a pink bowtie, so I bought some black paint and painted it black, but it's still drying."

I touched the bowtie and a black spot of paint dotted my finger. As a matter of fact, paint was dripping onto the floor and spots of smooth silky pink were appearing. I looked at my watch and thought it might be best to try to tie my original bowtie one more time. I went over to the trash and found the wastebasket was clean as a whistle.

Just my luck, they don't empty the trash for weeks and today some unseen trash gremlin decides to actually clean up a bit.

"Looks like I'm stuck with your black and pink bowtie, kid. Thanks for your troubles. I'll see you at the reception."

I hung up the tie in my makeshift changing room, over the sink and sat down for a few moments to collect my thoughts.

A bride who is eight and a half months pregnant, her mother fresh off the ship from the jungles of Africa, a wedding in a dilapidated store front medical clinic, the most motley crew of wedding guests one could ever imagine, and the prospect of spending the next thirty or forty years mending, prescribing, and caring for the dregs of society, is that what I really want? Look at them all; they look so happy, so excited and there is such an air of anticipation. I guess we really do some good work here. And, Miss James, lovely, wonderful Miss James, she truly is my anchor. Too late to change my mind, I guess it's on with the show.

I touched the bowtie and a new black spot on my finger appeared. I gingerly wiped off the back of the tie so that wet paint would not mar my shirt and then I snapped it in place. I bent over to put on my shoes and then I looked at myself in the mirror. Black paint adorned my chin, which I wiped off, most of it, anyway.

This won't work.

I took off the troublesome bowtie and wiped the all paint away, leaving a pink tie with a few black streaks. I rubbed and buffed until all the paint was either removed or dry.

Pink it is, I guess.

I admired myself in the mirror.

It looks pretty good, actually.

"Definitely your color," came a voice behind me. "Black tux with a shiny pink bowtie. If it was my poor Lizzy, may she rest in peace, she would have postponed the wedding until I found a proper tie, but Miss James is eminently more practical and will press on, I'm certain."

The voice belonged to Vince Smialdi, the clinic handyman and caretaker of Polly, an orange and purple dragon who had miraculously hatched at the Clinic one evening. Vince had agreed to be my best man, after my friend Max had to cancel on short notice for some fuzzy, vague reason.

"Where's Polly? You didn't bring her, did you?"

"What do you think? It's the Night Clinic crowd. You've got dwarves, vampires, werewolves, strippers, and the greatest assortment of bizarre characters this side of the rainbow. I don't think anyone will even blink over the site of a purple dragon. She's sitting with Roachman and Super Rat. They can look out for each other."

Vince came over to me and grabbed my hand and then gave me a hug. I looked him in the eye and saw the emotion.

"It looks like this is really going to happen," I concluded. "We've got a best man, a bride and groom, and the bride's mother. You've got the rings; I've got a pink bowtie and a spot of black paint on my chin which won't come off. All we need is the preacher."

It was almost time to begin and Pastor Horst hadn't made an appearance yet.

"Don't worry. I called him an hour ago and he promised he'd be here on time, awake, sober, and properly dressed," Vince reported.

"I don't suppose you asked him to take a bath and shave?" I added.

"Don't press it. One miracle at a time."

At that moment we heard the murmur of the crowd suddenly grow louder and then a loud crash.

"I guess we can stop worrying."

Sure enough, Pastor Gustav "Gussie" Horst had arrived in typical Horst fashion, surrounded by chaos and calamity. Vince looked out at the crowd and saw the pastor picking up a bucket and mop he had tripped over as part of his arrival.

"Looks like the pastor is functioning at his usual level. Let's hope he can make it through the ceremony upright and without dropping his Bible on anyone's foot or upsetting the podium. Why'd you pick him anyway?"

"Didn't have a lot of choice. It was short notice and we don't really have a regular preacher. Miss James thought it would be better to have someone from the community. He is ordained, after all..."

"Yeah, an ordained walking disaster. Look out there, I swear there is a black cloud over his head."

I looked out at the now full "chapel" and observed Pastor Horst standing in the makeshift pulpit and I saw the "black cloud." Hovering above Pastor Horst was the Raven, who circled around a few times and then took a position on one of the ceiling lights.

"That's not a cloud, Vince, it's a big black bird, one who was definitely not invited."

Vince grabbed a broom and started out to shoe the bird away.

"Don't bother," I informed him. "Even if you manage to get him out, which may not be that easy to do, he'll be back. He seems to like it here. Just leave him alone and there shouldn't be any problem."

I looked up at the clock, which read seven thirty.

"Well, here we go..."

I heard singing as Curley and Cupcake began:

> *He is now to be among you at the calling of your hearts*
> *Rest assured this troubador is acting on his part.*
> *The union of your spirits, here, has caused him to remain*
> *For whenever two or more of you are gathered in his name*
> *There is love. There is love.*

> *A man shall leave his mother and a woman leave her home*
> *And they shall travel on to where the two shall be as one.*
> *As it was in the beginning is now and til the end*
> *Woman draws her life from man and gives it back again.*
> *And there is love. There is love.*

> *Well then what's to be the reason for becoming man and wife?*
> *Is it love that brings you here or love that brings you life?*
> *And if loving is the answer, then who's the giving for?*
> *Do you believe in something that you've never seen before?*
> *Oh there's love, there is love.*

> *Oh the marriage of your spirits here has caused him to remain*
> *For whenever two or more of you are gathered in his name*
> *There is love. There is love.**

Before the song finished I made my way out to the altar and stood with Vince as we awaited the arrival of my bride. The lobby and waiting room almost made a respectable wedding chapel. Rows and rows of folding chairs took up almost all the floor space, leaving a narrow aisle down the middle. Pink and white carnations adorned the front where there was a wooden canopy above a small stage. There was a sign behind the altar, which read: "No spitting, urinating, or littering allowed in the lobby or waiting room" in big black and red letters, offering sharp contrast to the decorations.

Curley and Cupcake finished their song and new music began, a funky version of "Here Comes the Bride" courtesy of Wild Fingers Dixon on the guitar. I winked at Nurse James' mother, Betty James, who was seated in the front row dressed in her African kanga, and then I saw Miss James, more radiant than ever even with her big belly. She wore a light pink gown with white accents, spaghetti straps and a white veil.

Curley stood by her side, their arms intertwined, as she made her way down the aisle, doing her best to look solemn, but unable to hide her joy and happiness. Wild Fingers' melodious guitar heightened the mood as my bride drew closer. Just before Curley was to release her hand to join mine a buzz ran through the crowd as our guests began to point up at the ceiling.

I looked up and saw a pair of black wings flitting erratically between the lights.

The Raven? Another drunken bird? No, a bat.

The Raven, to its credit, took matters into its own hands and flew off its perch and gave chase. We all oohed and aahed as the two winged creatures bobbed and weaved between light fixtures and around vents. At first it looked like the Raven would easily dispatch the interloper, but then the bat would dodge one way or another and elude the black bird. The Raven made a final lunge at the bat and grabbed hold of its foot, but then the bat settled down in an empty chair and the Raven was left holding nothing but the pant leg of Mr. V.M. Pire.

"Sorry, I'm late," he explained, a bit sheepishly, "I had to wait until sundown. I'm sure you understand."

"Quite alright," I answered, "but you did ruin my lovely bride's entrance."

"Sorry," he said again and he stood and bowed. Everyone turned away from him, back towards the radiant Miss James. The Raven returned to his spot, perched above the gathering of guests, keeping a watchful eye over the ceremony.

The music resumed and Miss James made it to the altar without further trouble. I clasped her hand in mine as Curley took his seat between Cupcake and my soon to be mother-in-law.

Pastor Horst cleared his throat, "Hrrmph," took a deep breath and cleared his throat again, "Hrrrmmph." Then he coughed a few more times and finally stood facing us, his face even redder than usual.

"Dearly beloved," he began, "we are gathered here in the sight of God to join this man and this woman in holy matrimony, which is a holy estate ordained by God..."

I hope he's not too long winded. Just hit the high points and get this over with.

Hack... wheeze... cough.

And don't pass out.

At that moment a black cat jumped up on the altar.

OK, who brought the cat?

Daniel's dog, Becky, decided it was her job to rid the ceremony of uninvited felines and leapt up from the audience and dashed towards the cat and us.

"Rowf, Rowf, Grrr," barked Becky

"Meeoowww, meeeoowwww," the cat replied followed by a swipe at Becky's nose with her sharp claws.

"Rowf?" Becky replied. She stopped for a moment and then let out a long, "Grrrrr..."

The cat darted away into the crowd of guests and Becky followed, howling. Every so often there was a shout from one of our guests as the dog and cat weaved their way in and around chairs.

"Where did that cat come from?" Miss James wondered out loud.

"At the rate we're going, our daughter will have graduated medical school before we actually are married," I added.

Roachman came to the rescue, gathering up the cat and hustling it outside. Becky sniffed and barked at the door until she was sure the cat was gone and then took her place on the floor by Daniel's chair.

"This is highly irregular," Pastor Horst observed. "Such she-nanigans are not supposed to be part of such a solemn and auspicious occasion."

"It's OK Pastor. Believe me I wouldn't be surprised if the Wicked Witch of the West materialized right here in front of us."

At that moment there was a pillar of fire and green smoke right next to me. The smoke and fire dissipated leaving a figure dressed in a tight black dress, crooked pointed black hat, waving a broom and cackling. I looked up, questioning an unseen deity.

Is this really necessary?

"Who killed my sister, who killed the Wicked Witch of the East? Was it you?" she screamed at Miss James who found herself rubbing shoulders with the green-skinned witch.

My beloved opened her mouth, but no words came out and then I thought she was going to faint. I quickly moved to her side and put my arm around her, forcing myself between her and the Wicked Witch.

"There's no dead witch..." I started to explain, but then our own Wicked Queen, Queen of the strippers that is, approached her from behind.

"You're mistaken," she whispered in the real witch's ear. "Look around. There's no dead witch here. This is a place for healing and joy. We try to keep death away."

The Wicked Witch of the West did look around, all the time shaking her broomstick while cackling her distinctive laugh. Then she pulled up her black sleeve exposing her bony green arm and looked at her black watch and then she shook her wrist.

"Curses, curse that stupid spell. This isn't right. Where are the Munchkins? Where is that brat Dorothy or that goody two shoes Glinda. Let me check these instructions," she murmured as she pulled out a piece of faded brown paper. "Two eyes of newt, a rat tooth, a beagle's feather, boil for ten minutes and dip broom in..."

Curley decided he needed to add his two cents and got up from his seat, "Did you say 'beagle's feather, Ms. Witch?"

She nodded her head, "Yes, it says right here, 'beagle's feather.' "

Curley took the paper from her hand and put on his reading glasses. "If I read this correctly, Ms. Wicked Witch, it says 'an eagle's feather' not a 'beagle's feather.' The comma looks like a letter 'b'. Here check it for yourself. You can use my glasses if it will help."

The witch pulled out her own spectacles and perched them on her long, pointy green nose, and peered through them at the worn paper.

"Hmm, I guess you're right," she murmured scratching her chin. "It was no easy chore finding a beagle with feathers. I sort of had to improvise. Sorry for the interruption. You look lovely, my dear," she added speaking to Miss James and then she whispered, "stand back."

"Heh, heh, heh, heh," she cackled and she waved her broom, winked at us, and spun around as the pillar of green fire and smoke shot up from the floor and she vanished.

"Enough is enough," I said to no one in particular. "Let's get this show over with so we can really get down and party."

I looked for Pastor Horst, and found him, flat on the floor, unconscious. Together, Miss James and I knelt at his side. I felt for a pulse, while Miss James cradled his head.

"He's breathing," She observed.

"And he's got a strong radial pulse," I added.

He started to rouse and opened his eyes.

"What happened?" he wondered.

"As best as we can determine," Miss James answered, "you fainted."

"Is the wedding over?" he asked.

"We haven't really started yet," I replied. "But, we are ready whenever you are."

"OK, OK," he wheezed, "let's see if we can get you two married without further interruption."

He made it up to standing.

"Join hands, please," he requested of us. "Dearly beloved, we are gathered here today in the presence of God to join this man and this woman in holy matrimony, which is a blessed state."

He turned to me.

"Do you, Miles Standish Barnes, take this woman to be your lawful wedded wife? To have and to hold, to love and honor and cherish, in sickness and in health, until death do you part?"

"I do," I answered.

He turned towards Miss James.

"Do you, Portia Mathilda James, take this man to be your lawful wedded husband? To have and to hold, to love and honor and cherish, in sickness and in health, until death do you part?"

"I do," she answered and she stared into my eyes with more love than any man ever deserved.

"Is there a ring for our bride and groo..o...m..."

Pastor Horst's voice trailed off and he fell to the floor and began to snore.

"He's asleep," Vince observed

Narcolepsy? Why can't anything ever be simple?

Try as we could, we could not rouse the Pastor.

"I don't think we're married yet," Miss James remarked.

It was Madame Marie who came to the rescue.

"I'll finish the ceremony," she stated.

"Are you allowed, I mean would it be legal?" I asked, a bit skeptical.

"Of course, I am Voodoo High Priestess, fully licensed to perform a variety of religious functions."

I glanced over at Pastor Horst, who was snoring away on a mat on the floor in the corner and then at my bride. Miss James' eyes gave me her answer.

"OK, Madame, let's get this wedding done before our daughter decides she wants to be part of the ceremony."

So, Madame Marie took her place at the head of the altar. She reached into her bag and hung some feathers and a dead chicken from the canopy and the ceremony resumed.

"Who's got the ring?" she asked.

Vince handed the ring to Madame Marie, who held it up to the light and then took out a jeweler's loupe to examine it.

"Eighteen Karat gold with two and a half carat VVS, ideal cut G diamond, VS1, G color side stones, nice," she muttered under her breath and then she handed the ring to me.

"Place the ring on the fourth finger of her left hand and repeat after me," she commanded. " 'With this ring I thee wed.' "

"With this ring I thee wed," I repeated softly.

"And the other ring?"

Vince handed the second ring to Madame, who once again held it up to inspection.

"Pretty hefty, oh and it's engraved, also very nice," she smiled at me and handed the ring to Miss James. "Repeat after me, 'with this ring I thee wed.' "

"With this ring I thee wed," Miss James said staring into my eyes, her eyes saying so much more than the words.

"Therefore, by the powers vested in me by this great state, I now pronounce you husband and wife. May the magnificent Baron Samedi bless this union of souls. You may kiss the bride."

I gently put my arms around my dear Portia Barnes and kissed her.

"Miles and Portia Barnes? Perhaps we should keep it Dr. Barnes and Miss James," she whispered in my ear. I nodded my agreement.

The nuptials moved on to a grand and uneventful reception which featured music courtesy of Curley and Cupcake and Wild Fingers. Pastor Horst finally woke up and resumed his place among the living and had our guests in stitches with his rendition of a debate between Daffy and Donald Duck.

It was early morning when we finally found ourselves in the Bridal Suite at the Fairmont.

"It was a memorable night," I commented.

"You have a gift for understatement," Miss James replied. "Black cats, wicked witches, a voodoo high priestess? I'd say if we can survive a wedding like that, our marriage should be able to endure anything."

"Look at these gifts," I commented and I began to take inventory.

"Curley and Cupcake, *Play the Catskills: A Collection of Showtunes, Thirty Great Songs from Broadway and the Movies*."

"Just my style, hope it includes songs from *My Fair Lady*."

"Let's see, a used dirty cape with a big 'R' from Roachman; a gift certificate to 'The Enchanted Emporium.' "

"Not really my taste in entertainment."

"Evella, Goddess of the Night's recipe for butter cookies and brownies."

"Finally, something worthwhile, although I'll leave the baking to you."

"An ostrich foot from Madame Marie and a miniature version of... me."

"I'll take the doll, it'll help me keep you in line. I don't think you need the ostrich foot, however."

"You'll want this to go with the doll," I said and handed her a thin book, *Voodoo for Beginners*.

There were a lot more presents, ranging from cracked beer mugs someone probably swiped from a local bar to the occasional gift that actually would be useful such as a dinnerware for four and a set of satin sheets.

Finally I found the gift I'd been looking for. It was wrapped in plain brown paper which I tore off in great anticipation. Inside was a drawing, Caleb's gift to us. I held it up to the light and we both admired the extraordinary image he had created.

It showed the two of us, holding hands and walking together. We each carried a baby wrapped in a blanket as we walked over a river, only there wasn't any bridge. We were suspended in the sky, walking on beams of white and yellow light while below us was a raging river lined by sharp, jagged rocks. The source of lights could be seen far in the distance as we walked towards it. And, to add a bit of mystery or maybe peace of mind, a black bird flew overhead. The Raven.

The picture almost brought me to tears. I laid it against the wall.

"I know your eight and a half months pregnant, but maybe we can find a way to celebrate our wedding night?" I asked as I helped Portia undress.

"Where there's a will there's a way and, Dr. Barnes, I know you'll find it," she smiled and kissed me.

I opened my eyes and looked out the window. The Raven was perched on the ledge, but flew away as soon as I noticed it.

"Ooooh," Miss James moaned.

"Already?" I wondered out loud. "I've barely started."

"Aaaw, ooooh, I think..." she panted. "I think it's time."

"Anytime is right as far as I'm concerned," I answered and I gave her a letcherous look.

She took a few deep breaths.

"Oooh, Oooh... oh, yes, it's time, dear, wonderful, husband doctor. Time for the baby to arrive. Let's go."

So, we spent the rest of our wedding night having a beautiful baby girl.

*The Wedding Song, Noel "Paul" Stookey 1972

NIGHT CLINIC... FINALE?

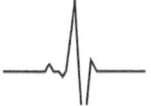

"DO YOU BELIEVE THIS? I MEAN THIS CAN'T BE TRUE," I raved as I read the article in the *Post*.

"City to Shutter Free Clinics
Council Cites Cost and Duplication of Services"

"You seem to be taking this rather calmly," I continued, addressing my dear wife, Nurse James.

She was preoccupied playing with our baby girl, Rose Elisabeth, who celebrated her three-month birthday that day.

"Happy Birthday, sweet Rose. Who's my big girl?" she cooed and held the girl up as high as she could reach.

Rose giggled and squealed.

"Forget the paper, at least for a while. Just look at this smile, this big beautiful smile."

I did put the paper down and stood behind my two girls.

It will be OK. Just remember this is what is truly important. But, our patients? They're important, too.

"I suppose you're right, it will work out for the best. But, how many of our patients will be able to be cared for at the University Clinic? Walking two or three blocks is a lot different than taking a bus across town."

"They'll never close *our* Clinic. We do too much good work," she concluded.

"All the politicians care about is dollars, mostly how much they can put in their own pockets. You know what I always say..."

"Yes, yes, they are only two types of politicians, those that are in jail for corruption and those who haven't been caught yet."

"I'm glad you pay attention. Let me look at page eight where they go into more specifics about the clinics slated to be closed."

Pages rustled and Rose laughed as I found the rest of the article.

"The free clinics which are to be closed have not yet been determined, but speculation is that clinics in neighborhoods where there is access to other care, such as private Urgent Care clinics and free standing Emergency Rooms will be the first on the chopping block..."

"See, we should be OK. There certainly are none of those in that part of town."

"There's more. 'In addition, those clinics in parts of the city where the crime rate is high or there is an unusual amount of gang activity also may be shuttered. Public hearings, where private citizens may voice their concerns, will be held in the next few weeks. Exact time and venue will be announced.' I think *that* means we're in trouble."

Miss James stared at Rose and then held her close to her chest. Rose instinctively tried to help herself to a snack.

"Well," Miss James began, "we've got a few weeks anyway. We should plan to go to those hearings. You know, speak up for the downtrodden."

"You're right, like always," I answered as I looked at the clock. "Six thirty? I better be on my way. I hope there isn't much traffic or I'll be late. I don't want to ruin my perfect record."

Miss James smiled at me and my "perfect record," but didn't comment. I kissed Rose and my lovely wife.

"I wish it was next week and you were back at work," I commented as I gathered up my white coat. "The other nurses are OK, but they are not Nurse James."

I began the usual thirty-minute drive to the Clinic.

Not too much traffic for a change. I can't believe they would even think about closing our clinic. On the other hand, if we have to move, maybe we'll find a proper medical facility with a real modern lab and state of the art imaging. Dream on, Doctor. This is not Beverly Hills or Beacon Hill. As far as politicians are concerned: no money, no voice. Then again, maybe I shouldn't be so cynical. Here I am entering the "clinic neighborhood" and it's not so bad. There are some trees over here and a little park. And, on the corner, members of one of our many independent youth groups are hanging out. There's even some new construction going up. It's hard to believe, but someone, somewhere, actually has an interest in developing this part of town. Funny, I don't know why I never noticed it before. Whatever that building's going to be, it looks very elaborate.

My head shifted away from my troubles as the radio blasted out some classic rock:

Sitting on a park bench
Eyeing little girls with bad intent... hey Aqualung

Jethro Tull seems very appropriate for this part of town.

I arrived at 6:55 and was greeted by Miss James' sub, Mrs. Selma Cranston. She looked exactly like one would expect someone named Selma Cranston would look, mid fifties, matronly, dull brown hair tied back into a bun, adorned with a white, knee length dress, white stockings and white shoes.

I'm surprised she isn't wearing a white nurse's cap.

"Good evening, Dr. Barnes, I'm Mrs. Cranston. I'll be helping you tonight. This is my first night here and I've never been in a clinic *like this*, so I hope you'll be patient."

"Glad to meet you. I'm sure you'll do fine. It's a bit of work, because it's just the two of us. No techs, no aids, but we usually manage."

What did she mean, "clinic like this?" We're just like any other clinic; that is if those other clinics are visited by Ravens, bizarre superheroes, vampires, werewolves, and mythological beasts.

"There's a patient in Room One, Milo Campo, 63, complaining of a non-healing wound. He's wearing a pith helmet and carrying a toy rifle. Oh, and I brought some fried chicken to eat, in case you get hungry later."

"From Purdy's Chicken Shack?"

"Where else?"

Mrs. Cranston just moved up a few notches on my approval rating scale.

"Well, then let's get to work," I replied.

I picked up the chart for Mr. Campo. Non-healing wound on right buttock, no allergies, travelled to Tanzania recently, no other medical problems.

I did my usual quick knock and went in.

"Good evening, Mr. Campo. What is the problem which brought you into our fine Clinic this evening."

"Get down, get down or he'll get away," he hissed through clenched teeth.

I looked back over my shoulder and then around the room.

"Who or what will get away," I wondered out loud.

"The rhino, of course. Now get down before you get trampled."

This can't be happening.

Mr. Campo was dressed in beige safari gear, sported a gray pith helmet, and was carrying a large, plastic hunter's rifle. He grabbed me by the arm and pulled my arm, with considerable force, I must add. I joined him crouching behind the exam table.

"I don't see the rhino," I whispered.

He handed me his glasses.

"They asked me to check your wound, the one on your buttock," I said. "How did you get it and when?" I added.

He looked around, pointed his toy rifle but then put it back at his side. He put his mouth against my ear.

"I was attacked by a rhino, a rare, vicious black beast who gored me in the buttock with his horn almost a year ago," He replied in a very low monotone. "But, I'm on the trail of that black demon. It's not just any old rhino, you know. The monster I'm trailing is the rare Sumatran Three Headed Rhino. That's right, three heads, three horns, and a heart as black as its hide. When I get the rhino's three horns, I'll grind them up and sprinkle some of the dust on my wound. Its special properties will make it heal in a few days. The rest of the dust will be saved for the future. One can't be too careful or unprepared these days."

I nodded my head in agreement.

"Speaking of wounds," I countered. "I believe you are here to have that wound checked, by a doctor, specifically, Dr. Barnes, who is me?"

"Oh, yeah, right. I've lost the trail anyway, Dr. Barnes."

"Well, just drop your jeans and I'll take a look."

Mr. Campo slid his beige khaki pants and underwear down to his knees revealing a wound on his right cheek which was open to the air, about twelve by ten centimeters, extending into the subcutaneous tissue, but not involving any muscle or bone. There was some yellowish drainage, but no redness.

"How do you take care of this?" I queried.

"Take care of? I just leave it alone. It doesn't hurt. I just have to change my underwear every few days."

"Well, I think," I began, "if you cared for it properly and kept a bandage on it, perhaps it might start to..."

"There it goes," my patient screamed, "you won't get away, you brute."

And, Mr. Campo burst out of the Exam Room, trying to run while pulling up his underwear and pants at the same time. It was all I could do to hold the laughter inside as he finally got his pants pulled up and fastened and then bounded away, chasing his imaginary, three headed rhinoceros.

Oh, well, you lose some and then you lose some. Onward to new frontiers.

I moved on to Room Two, Myron Davis, 38, complaining of abdominal pain for five days. No previous medical problems, no allergies, no meds.

Should be simple.

"Good evening, Mr. Davis, what brings you into our Night Clinic?" I began.

Myron Davis was dressed in a black suit, white shirt with French cuffs, blue paisley tie, black socks, and shiny, black leather shoes. He definitely did not have the look of our usual client. He was half sitting, half laying in the chair, his black hat perched on his chest, and did not get up to greet me. His face was flushed and beads of sweat dotted his forehead.

"Hiya Doc, I hope you can help me," he replied to my introduction. He looked around the room as if he there were other people present.

"It's just you and me, Mr. Davis. Now what seems to be bothering you?"

"It's my gut, Dr....Barnes," he answered staring at my name tag. "It feels like someone is driving a metal stake through it."

"When did this pain begin?" I asked.

"Twenty years ago."

"Did you say twenty years? Why did you come in tonight?"

"Excuse me, Dr. Barnes, but are you recording this?"

"No," I responded truthfully.

"Is any of what I say going into any sort of database or computer?"

"No, I'll write it down and it will go into a chart."

"A written chart, nothing electronic?"

"Sorry, to disappoint you, Mr. Davis, but we are not a very well funded clinic. Computers and IPads cost money; money the taxpayers apparently are loathe to spend. So, here we are, paper, pens, stone knives, and bearskins."

"That's good, very good," he concluded. "They won't be able to find me."

"Excuse me?" I had to ask. "But, who won't be able to find you?"

"The spies, the government, our government, the Russians, the Germans, the Japanese, the Chinese, insurance companies, credit bureaus, credit card companies, banks, Disney; they're all spying on us, spying on me, all the time, watching every move you and I make, watching every moment of our lives with massive computers."

"Are you sure about this?"

"No question. Tell me, if someone makes an unauthorized purchase with your American Express card, do you get an e-mail or text message or phone call? Or, maybe all three. How do they know?"

"Hmmm…" was my reply, "but what about your abdom…?"

"Don't trust anyone is my creed. No credit cards, no bank account, no social security number, just pay cash for everything, leave no digital footprint and no one will knock on your door in the middle of the night and cart you off to CIA headquarters."

"Your abdominal pain," I tried again to get a history. "When does it occur?"

He looked at me and then at his stomach and then took a deep breath.

"I began with this pain about twenty years ago when all this computer stuff started to grow. It was the World Wide Web which made me realize that no matter what I do, someone, somewhere is going to find out or be affected. Then it was online banking and credit cards and MySpace then Facebook and Twitter. But I learned the truth. Someone is always watching, always monitoring. I couldn't find any peace. Sleep has become a luxury I just can't afford. What if I say something about my pain? Someone will be listening. Well, my pain has just stayed with me. So, I took a chance and went to see doctors. I tried Tagamet, then Zantac, Prilosec, antacids. I had EGD's and gallbladder surgery and finally resigned myself to my throwaway diagnosis: IBS."

"So," I interjected, "why are you here tonight?"

"Oh, I need some meds refilled. If I call a pharmacy to get my prescription refilled they'll put it in their computer and that'll be the end. *They* will know where I am."

"So all you want are some free samples? That's easy. If we have any, you are welcome to them."

"Just Carafate, it's the only thing which helps."

"Give me a minute and I'll check in the back."

"Uh, what are you writing?"

"Just your diagnosis and treatment. Probable gastritis, treat with Carafate. Samples given."

"But, didn't you hear anything I said. Everybody's watching, they'll find out. Sure, you only write it down now, but next month someone scans that chart and then, boom, I won't be able to get health insurance, find a job, anything. I'll be labeled, branded for life with... just the sound of it is ominous... gas-tri-tis. A mixture of gas and garbage. Just forget I was ever here. And, please, shred that chart."

Mr. Davis got up, put on his fine black hat and walked out.

Two for two. A great start to the night.

"Room Three," I murmured. "Misty Rowe, ten, fever, cough, history of leukemia. No allergies."

I knocked and went in starting my intro before I even saw my patient's face.

"Good evening, Mis..." I started, but stopped when I was greeted by Evella, Goddess of the Night.

"Dr. Barnes, congratulations," she said softly, her voice a bit raspy.

"Thank you, Evella, Goddess of the Night," I answered, but I was a bit shocked at her appearance. In the three months since I'd last seen her at my wedding, she had wasted away. Her skin was now a pasty yellow and her eyes almost glowed with jaundice. But, she still had her smile and her feisty demeanor.

"This is Misty, Dr. Barnes, a friend of mine. We met at the hospital while we were being treated. She's in remission from ALL. Her mother works nights a lot and I watch her when I'm well enough. I do have a consent from her mother so that I can make medical decisions for Misty, if you're worried about the legal niceties."

"No, no, I'm sure everything is in order," I said softly, a bit distracted by Evella's cachectic appearance. I recovered my composure and added, "What's the problem, Misty?"

"I've got a bad cough and my chest hurts. My fever today was 102.8."

"Have you been treated for your leukemia recently?"

"My last chemo was four months ago. I thought I just had a cold, but Miss Worry Wart here insisted we come to see you."

I listened to her chest, which was clear, inspected and palpated, shot a chest X-Ray which was normal, diagnosed her with a cold, and gave instructions for her to call her Pediatrician and Oncologist the next day.

I'm more worried about Evella.

"Misty, if you don't mind," I asked my young patient, "I'd like to talk with Evella, the Goddess of the Night, alone."

"You don't have to worry about me, Dr. Barnes," she answered. "I know she's got bad cancer and I know she's probably not going to live much longer. Just like my friends, Justin and Liv. They died of their cancer. I cried for them, but, at least they didn't have to suffer very long."

"Kids with cancer live with death hanging over their head every day," Evella explained. "You're a doctor, you should know that. Anyway, anything you have to say, you may say in front of Misty. We have no secrets and she knows I'm dying. I assume that's what you wanted to talk about."

"Such remarkable intuition, Evella, Goddess of the Night, of course that's what I want to talk about. Our first meeting taught me more about healing and the proper way to be a physician than all the lectures and rounds combined. And, you make great cookies. I'll miss them and you."

"You're sweet, Dr. Barnes," she said in that special voice she had as she patted me on the cheek and then on my derriere. "However, even though this vile cancer has had the gall to invade most of my vital organs, I am not planning to check out as soon as everyone thinks. I've got a lot of years of livin' to pack into the time I have left. See this?"

She held up a colorful brochure.

"Two week cruise in the Mediterranean. Barcelona, Monte Carlo, Venice, Rome, Athens, all the food I can eat, first class all the way. If I'm going out, I'm going out in style."

"Sounds great," I observed. "You don't need a companion, do you? Because, the news is that this place may be shut down which will leave me out of a job."

"You're still sweet, but not my type. Don't worry about me, I'll find some young buck to keep me company."

"I wish you nothing but the best, Goddess," I added.

I gave her a kiss on the cheek and, at that moment, we heard music coming from the lobby. The familiar strains of "Night Clinic Blues" no doubt being strummed by the talented hands of Wild Fingers.

Two in the morning? Very strange, very strange indeed.

We all went out to the lobby where Wild Fingers Dixon sat strumming his guitar, softly humming along. There were a few patients waiting to be seen and they seemed to appreciate the early morning concert.

"...Oh Night Clinic Blues..."

A familiar bluesy voice joined the guitar.

"Dear Nurse James, what are you doing here at," I looked at my watch, "two eighteen in the morning and who's watching the baby?"

"She's here with me. Neither one of us could sleep and she kept pining away to see her father, so what could I do?"

She held little Rose up and I gave both my girls a big kiss.

"You do your work and all of us will keep Rose entertained," she decided. "Good evening, Evella and..."

"This is Misty, a friend of mine who wasn't feeling well, but, your wonderful husband has made us both feel better," Evella answered.

"I'm not so sure of that," I replied "and, if you'll excuse me, I have a few more sick people to see."

I left them in the lobby as Wild Fingers shifted to "God Bless the Child," one of my favorites. I listened for the deep soulful voice of my wife while perusing the chart of my next patient.

Elsa Waldenstein, 78, deaf, complaining of severe headache.

I hope she brought an interpreter.

I knocked and went in to Room One. Fortunately, there was a younger woman seated with my patient.

"Good evening, I'm Dr. Barnes. What's the problem you are having?"

The older woman sat in her chair and stared at me with a smile on her face, but it was obvious she did not comprehend. She was wearing a light jacket which covered her thin short dress, slightly worn white tights, and square-toed ballet slippers.

"Hello to you, Dr. Barnes," the younger woman replied. "My name is Eva Schosser and this is my mother, Elsa Waldenstein. She has been having headaches for about three weeks and they seem to be getting worse. I'm sorry she can't tell you herself. She's almost totally deaf and only speaks German."

Eva was middle aged, neatly dressed, with light brown hair and blue eyes which revealed only concern and worry.

"Why did you decide to bring her here tonight?" I queried.

"She told me that her headache was much worse and she felt like someone was pounding on the inside of her head with an ax."

"That's how she described it? Pounding with an ax?"

"Yes. Does that mean something?"

"Probably not, but it is an interesting choice of words."

"How's her health in general?"

"Considering her tortured past, excellent."

"Tortured past?"

"Dr. Barnes, Elsa Waldenstein was famous in the old country. She was on her way to becoming Prima Ballerina for the top ballet company in East Germany. Unfortunately, one of the party officials took an unusual interest in her, a very intimate and unnatural interest. The rest of the story is not pretty. Let's just say that she escaped East Germany and came to this country with nothing except the clothes on her back and a baby growing inside. Her flight to freedom was arduous with danger constantly lurking, but she survived and made it to this country. Unfortunately, there was a price. Hardship and injury caused her to lose her hearing, thus ending her dance career. She was granted political asylum here, but has lived a very hard and difficult life. A deaf woman with a newborn baby who doesn't speak the language has few prospects. But, we survived. Only now she has these headaches and she cannot find rest. I'm afraid for her; afraid that this relentless malady will finally break her spirit."

An amazing story.

"I will certainly do my best to help her," I said hoping both Eva and Elsa sensed the genuine concern in my voice. "Let me examine her now."

I started at the top and worked my way down. Everything was normal. As a matter of fact, she appeared remarkably healthy for a 78-year-old woman.

"Was she doing anything unusual when the headaches began? Or, has she suffered any injury, even something very minor?"

"Not that I'm aware of, but I'll ask."

Asking Elsa a question involved a complex series of hand gestures and written notes in German, which were followed by head shaking, nodding, more notes, and finally, calm.

"She says no," was the final result.

"I wish we had a CT Scanner, but we're just a poorly-equipped community clinic. Let me try something. I'll be back in a minute."

I asked Mrs. Cranston to start an IV on Elsa and then took care of the other two patients who were waiting, both with simple problems which were easily treatable with medications. They were sent on their way and I returned to Elsa and Eva.

"I've got something here that I think will help Elsa's headache," I explained to Eva. "It's some medicine that will relieve any tension she may have in her muscles. It works almost immediately."

"Thank you, Dr. Barnes," Eva said and then she wrote a message to Elsa who looked up at me with hope in her eyes.

I took a syringe from my pocket and injected one milligram of Versed through her IV. She winced a little when it first went in.

Eva and I watched as the forlorn look on Elsa's face began to fade. She closed her eyes and then the corners of her mouth began to turn up and a smile appeared. She opened her eyes and I saw a twinkle of life appear which had been absent just a few seconds earlier. She jumped up from her chair and took off her coat, revealing her light dress and dancer's body. She took my hand lightly and caressed it and then she did a pirouette.

"I think the medicine has helped," I observed.

But there was more. She exited the Exam Room and when she saw Wild Fingers with his guitar she gestured for him to play. She stared at his fingers as he started to play, a classical piece which I didn't recognize. Elsa, however, saw something that must have been from her past.

She began to dance, *en pointe*, moving gracefully across the waiting room on her toes, jumping and spinning in perfect rhythm to the music. The first rays of the sunrise pierced the Clinic windows creating a dazzling display of colors and illuminating Elsa in an array of red, orange, yellow, green, blue, and purple. She danced to me and curtsied, she elegantly leapt over chairs and spun around tables as those of us in audience stood in awe and applauded.

But, it could not last. The beautiful display was interrupted by three men, dressed in three black suits, wearing three pairs of black rimmed glasses, and carrying three identical black briefcases.

This has to be bad news.

"Doctor," man number one began, "I am Mr. Jacobs from the Department of Health. This is Mr. Binder from the City Inspector's Office and that is Mr. Berkowitz representing City council. May we talk to you?"

Jacobs, Binder and Berkowitz. Perfect name for a law firm.

"Certainly," I answered. "We can talk here."

"Is there some place more private?" one of three inquired.

"Anything you have to say, you may say here, as I'm sure it may have some effect on my patients.

Wild Fingers, Evella and Misty, who was holding Rose, Eva and Elsa, and Mrs. Cranston all stood silently, anticipating bad news. Miss James had vanished.

"As you wish," black suit number three answered. "We have an order here for this Clinic to be vacated immediately. It is the conclusion of the City Inspector's office that this building is unsafe and poses a hazard to anyone who occupies it. City Council has voted that this Clinic be closed immediately. We are now requesting that the premises be vacated immediately."

"But, Mr... uh... Berkowitz, what will become of the people who live in this neighborhood, who depend on this Clinic for their well being, where will they go?"

"Doctor, I'm sure your intentions are most noble, but this building is unsafe. Would you want to be examining a sick child and have the building collapse? Of course not. All of your patients will be more than welcome at the County Hospital Clinic."

"County? That's five miles away. Do you expect our patients to walk?"

"Doctor... Barnes, I will not argue any further. The decision has been made. This building will be demolished and County Hospital will assume the care of your patients."

"I won't leave. I'm staying right here." Defiant words came from behind me, from Miss James. "You'll have to cut my arm off to get me to move."

At that moment there was a faint "click" and my dear wife handcuffed herself to a sink which was behind the reception desk.

"Misty, if you could please hand me baby Rose. Thank you."

And, there we were, a standoff. On the one side were three carbon copy bureaucrats waving legal papers and, on the other, Miss James and Rose, battling for the little people. I was putting my money on my wife and baby.

The three men looked at each and then at Miss James and then at each other again.

I think she may actually win.

A voice interrupted the confrontation.

"THERE IT IS, THAT THREE HEADED MONSTER," it shouted. Milo Campo returned.

"I've finally tracked it down after all this time. You won't get away from me this time you vicious rhino. Black as night with a black heart to match. You'll pay for what you did to me."

"That's a real rifle he's pointing," I whispered to Evella, who was standing close to me. Maybe we should get down."

She nodded and we both stated to lower ourselves to the floor, as did the others in attendance.

My wife and Rose, they're stuck.

"Prepare to pay," Mr. Campo hissed through clenched teeth as he pulled the trigger.

Shots were fired and then there was a short scream. I jumped up and shielded Miss James and Rose, just in time to see Elsa jump, pirouette, and push Jacobs, Binder, and Berkowitz out of harm's way. Evella tried to tackle Mr. Campo as he kept shooting, only now his rifle was pointing harmlessly at the ceiling, knocking out the lights and setting off the sprinkler system. Finally, the shooting stopped as Wild Fingers and Evella wrestled the gun away.

There was another scream as Eva knelt beside Elsa, who was lying in pool of blood.

I ran to her side as sirens whined in the distance.

Misty hung up the phone and shouted, "Ambulance and police are on the way."

I felt a very thready pulse on Elsa as she smiled at me, struggling to breathe.

"Good doctor," she whispered to me in English.

The pulse vanished.

I started CPR, but Eva stopped me.

"Please," she said, "Please, don't; you gave her a few minutes of peace and joy, but let her go. Just remember; remember the smile on her face and remember her dancing."

Eva looked at her mother's lifeless face and buried her face in her chest. Tears streamed down her cheeks when she looked up.

You know," she began, trying to speak through her tears, "I had never seen her dance before. Oh, I'd seen newspaper clippings and photos in her scrapbook, but never the real thing. You gave me a gift that will be with me forever. And, I will be able to watch her happiness over and over."

She had recorded her mother's dance on her phone and now the graceful beauty of that dance would live forever on YouTube.

The police came and took Mr. Campo away in handcuffs. Jacobs, Binder, and Berkowitz left their papers with the day shift crew who started to appear and begin the task of moving everything out. The police cordoned off where the shooting had occurred and went through the motions of performing an investigation. I resigned myself to looking for a new work venue.

My dear Miss James, however, remained defiant.

"Call the papers, call channel twelve," she screamed. "I can see the headlines: 'Bureaucrats Try to Oust Mother and Baby.' All the publicity will surely keep us open."

"Are you sure about this?" I asked. "Is this what's right for Rose?"

This cannot end well.

But, our luck was about to change.

I heard a car screech to a stop outside the Clinic and looked up to see a big black limousine.

Even more trouble?

A burly chauffeur stepped out and opened the rear door. Out stepped a woman dressed in pink, bright pink which shimmered as the morning sun outlined her perfect figure. A broad white hat and dark glasses shielded her face. There was the sparkle of emerald and diamond earrings and emerald and diamond rings adorning her perfect beauty. As this mystery woman walked closer, ignoring the police barricade, I realized I knew her.

Medusa.

I looked up at the sky and was not disappointed as Pegasus circled overhead. There was a faint whinny as that noble equine acknowledged me.

"Medusa…" I began, but she held up her hand.

She gave me a light kiss on my cheek as I took her hand and led her into the Clinic lobby where she removed the hat and sun-glasses, allowing her long silky hair to fall about her shoulders. She was even more beautiful than I remembered.

"I see you've moved up in the world," I observed.

"My life is a rollercoaster. The fruit of immortality, I suppose. He's good to me, fun and rich and generous. Which is why I'm here."

"You're going to make a donation to the Dr. Barnes Survival and Party Fund?" I asked facetiously.

She looked me in the eye and then answered, "Not quite, but close. Have you seen the new building going up a few blocks over? The fancy one?"

"Yeah, I was wondering what it was going to be."

"That, dear Dr. Barnes, is going to be your new home, that is, the new Clinic. I read about the budget cuts and I was worried that this Clinic might be in line to get the ax."

I was speechless for a moment and then I said a soft, "Thank you."

"No," she replied, "Thank you."

"Me?"

She looked down at the floor and then stared into my eyes again.

"I was cold and you made me warm," she explained. "For that simple act of kindness I am grateful. And for all the acts of kindness you and the people at this Clinic perform, we are all grateful and indebted to you."

She reached into her Hermes purse and fumbled around for a

moment before pulling out a big manila envelope."

"Here are all the details. There is an endowment of $150 million to keep the Clinic funded. The new Clinic will have a larger waiting room, eight Exam Rooms, a Procedure Room, a complete Lab which will be properly staffed, Radiology with a CT Scanner and ultrasound, also staffed, a kitchen, storage, and doctor's offices. You also have my pledge that you will not want for anything as long as I'm alive, which, as you know, will be a long time."

"I don't know how to thank you, for myself and all the people who live here. When will it be ready?"

"About two months from now."

"And between now and then?"

"You're stuck here, I'm afraid."

"But, the building's been deemed unsafe; we're supposed to vacate."

"Ah, yes, that. Politics and graft. My husband did some checking. Some of our less scrupulous political servants were trying to get this space at a cut rate price. They bribed a City Inspector to condemn the building so that they could put up some sort of shopping mall or low rent housing or something. Whatever, they'll be on their way to jail soon."

"Did you hear all that, Miss James?" I turned to my wife, still handcuffed to the sink. "I guess you can set yourself free."

"Yes, it all sounds wonderful," Miss James answered. "Now, if you'll just get me the key, I'll set myself free."

"The key? What key?" I asked.

"The key in the desk in the back. It's where you keep your stuff. I found these cuffs back there and came up with the idea to chain myself to the building."

"I'll go look, but I've never seen those handcuffs before. In the meantime, maybe Medusa would like to see beautiful baby Rose?"

I took Rose from my wife and handed her to Medusa and went into the back to find the key. I searched high and low, up and down, back and forth, but there was no key. I had no choice but to report my failure and suffer Miss James wrath.

"WHAT, NO KEY? DO YOU EXPECT ME TO STAY CHAINED TO THIS TOILET FOREVER?"

"It's a sink," I corrected.

She tried to kick me. Medusa once again came to my rescue.

"I think I can help," she offered, "rather, Pegasus can help."

"What can a horse do about handcuffs?" Miss James wondered, showing a distinct lack of faith and understanding of things mythological.

"I'm game to try anything," I added.

Medusa let out a loud long whistle and Pegasus alighted outside the Clinic door. Medusa whispered in his ear and he turned around so that his hindquarters faced my wife.

"Close your eyes," Medusa commanded.

Miss James and I both closed our eyes. There was a sharp noise as Pegasus gave a precise kick and the handcuffs opened up.

Miss James rubbed her wrists as she got up and bowed before the winged horse.

"Thank you, both of you," she addressed Medusa and Pegasus. "I wish you both a long and happy life."

I also thanked them and walked Medusa to her limousine.

"Will we see each other again?" I wondered out loud.

"Perhaps, should the opportunity or need arise. I have a special place in my heart for you. The envelope I left has the name of the builder and architect for your new clinic. Good luck and be happy," she advised as she climbed into her fancy limo and drove away.

"Rose," I said, holding up my daughter, "I think you are due for a change. A diaper change."

Miss James and I carried her to the back.

"And, just what were you doing with handcuffs?" she asked as she grabbed my arm.

"Me, I thought they were yours," I answered. "What could I possibly do with a pair of handcuffs?"

"I can think of a few things," Miss James remarked as she bent over to change Rose's diaper, trying to hide the smirk on her face, while presenting a perfect view of her shapely bottom.

About the Author

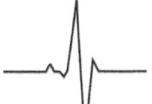

DAVID GELBER, A NEW YORK NATIVE, IS THE SEVENTH OF nine sons and one of three to pursue medicine. He graduated from Johns Hopkins University in 1980 and went on to graduate medical school in 1984 from the University of Rochester.

He completed a residency in General Surgery at Baylor University Medical Center in Dallas, TX, and Nassau County Medical Center on Long Island, NY, in 1989. Dr. Gelber now is in private practice in Houston, TX.

Gelber has been performing surgery for more than 25 years, but over the last few years he began to pursue his passion for writing, initially with his debut novel, *Future Hope*, followed by its sequel *Joshua and Aaron*.

These were followed by two books about surgery, *Behind the Mask* and *Under the Drapes*. The apocalyptic, *Last Light*, and historical fantasy, *Minotaur Revisited*, round out his published works, while numerous articles have appeared on his blog, "Heard in the OR."

Now he presents *Little Bit's Story*, and his collection of magical medical short stories, *Night Clinic*, will soon be released.

He has been married to Laura for 28 years and has three college-aged children. He and Laura share their home with five dogs and numerous birds.

Books Published

Future Hope
ITP Book One

Joshua and Aaron
ITP Book Two

Minotaur Revisited

Behind the Mask:
The Mystique of Surgery and the Surgeons who Perform Them

Under the Drapes: More Mystique of Surgery

Last Light (e-book only)

Blog:

Heard in the OR
http://heardintheor.blogspot.com